# Table of Contents

## Chapter 9 : Vegan



## Chapter 10 : Beverages



## Chapter 11 : Healthy Fish and Shellfish

- Staying Motivated on a Diabetic Diet

- Frequently Asked Questions

- Tips and Meal Plans

# Chapter 1: Introduction

## Welcome to Soul Food for Diabetics

Welcome to "Soul Food Cookbook for Diabetics," a culinary journey that brings together the rich, comforting flavors of traditional soul food with the health-conscious adaptations needed for managing diabetes. This book is a celebration of culture, tradition, and well-being, proving that you can enjoy your favorite dishes without compromising your health.

## The Importance of Soul Food in Culture and Tradition

Soul food is more than just a cuisine; it's a testament to resilience, creativity, and community. Rooted in the African American experience, soul food embodies a rich history of making the most out of limited resources, turning simple ingredients into hearty, flavorful meals. These dishes are often associated with family gatherings, celebrations, and cherished memories, making them an integral part of cultural identity.

## Adapting Soul Food for a Diabetic-Friendly Diet

Managing diabetes doesn't mean giving up on the foods you love. It means making smart choices and thoughtful adaptations. In this cookbook, we've reimagined classic soul food recipes to be lower in sugar, salt, and unhealthy fats, while still preserving the delicious flavors and satisfying textures that make soul food so beloved. Each recipe is designed to help you maintain stable blood sugar levels, support heart health, and nourish your body.

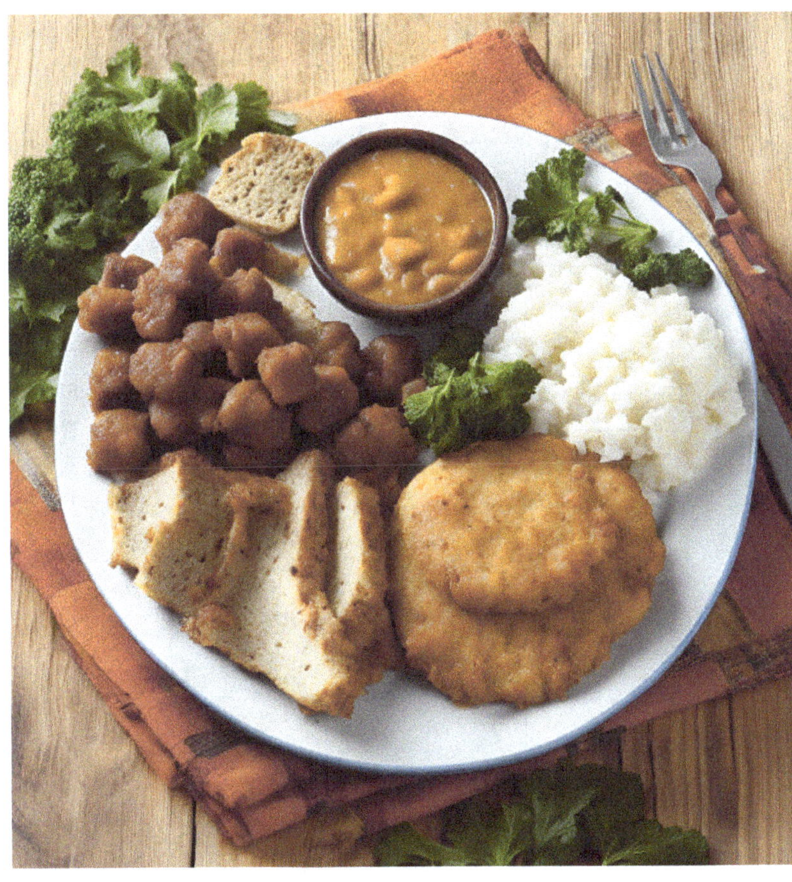

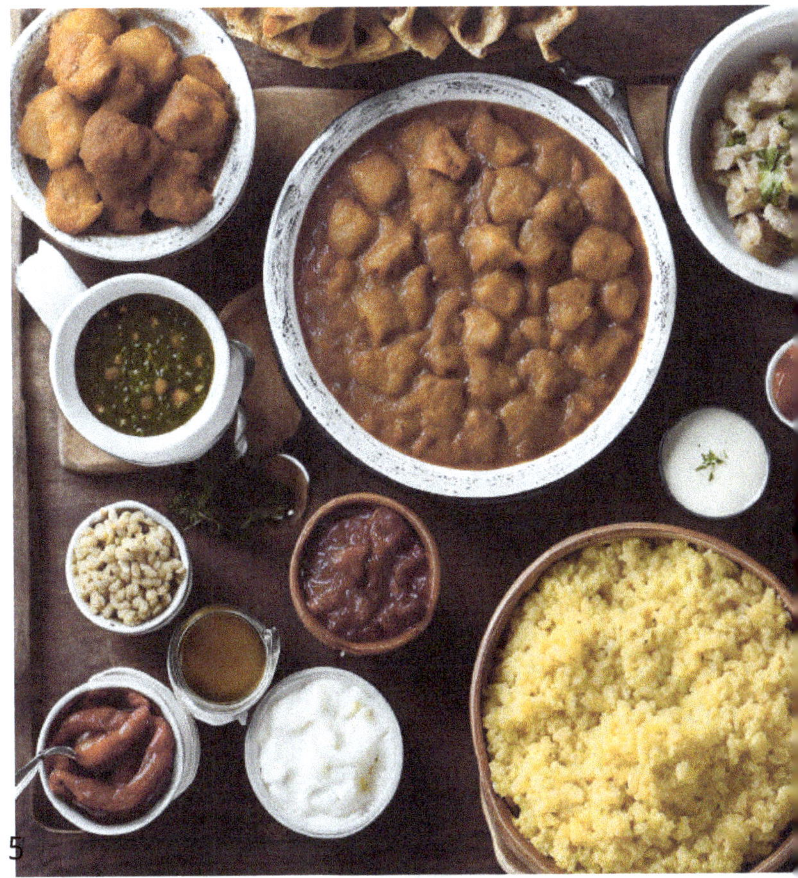

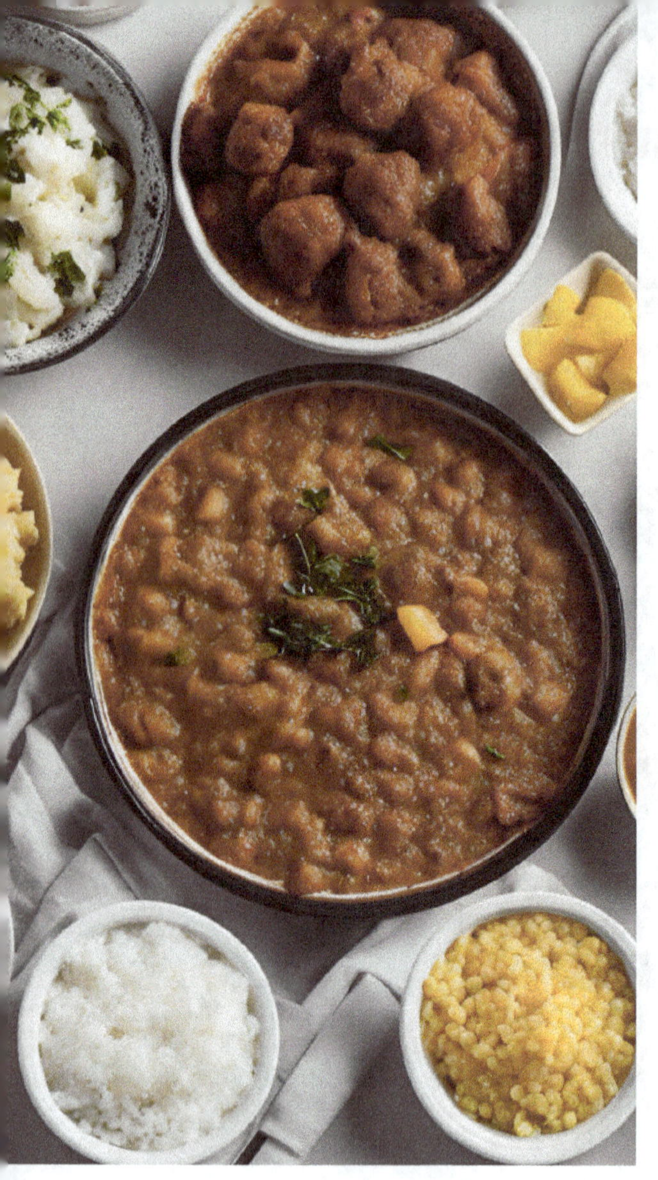

**Tips for Managing Diabetes through Diet**

**1. Monitor Carbohydrate Intake:** Pay attention to the types and amounts of carbohydrates you consume. Opt for complex carbohydrates like whole grains, vegetables, and legumes that provide sustained energy and have a lower impact on blood sugar levels.

**2. *Balance Your Plate:*** Aim for a balanced plate with a variety of nutrients. Fill half your plate with non-starchy vegetables, a quarter with lean protein, and the remaining quarter with whole grains or starchy vegetables.

**3. *Choose Healthy Fats:*** Incorporate healthy fats from sources like olive oil, avocados, nuts, and fatty fish. These fats can help improve heart health and provide essential nutrients.

**4. *Limit Added Sugars and Sodium:*** Reduce your intake of added sugars and sodium. Use herbs, spices, and natural sweeteners like stevia or monk fruit to enhance flavor without compromising your health.

**5. *Stay Hydrated:*** Drink plenty of water throughout the day. Staying hydrated helps regulate blood sugar levels and supports overall health.

**6. *Practice Portion Control:*** Be mindful of portion sizes to avoid overeating. Using smaller plates and bowls can help control portions and prevent excessive calorie intake.

**By following these tips and embracing the delicious recipes in this cookbook, you can enjoy the comforting flavors of soul food while taking control of your health. Let's embark on this journey together, savoring every bite and celebrating the vibrant traditions of soul food in a way that supports a healthy, balanced lifestyle.**

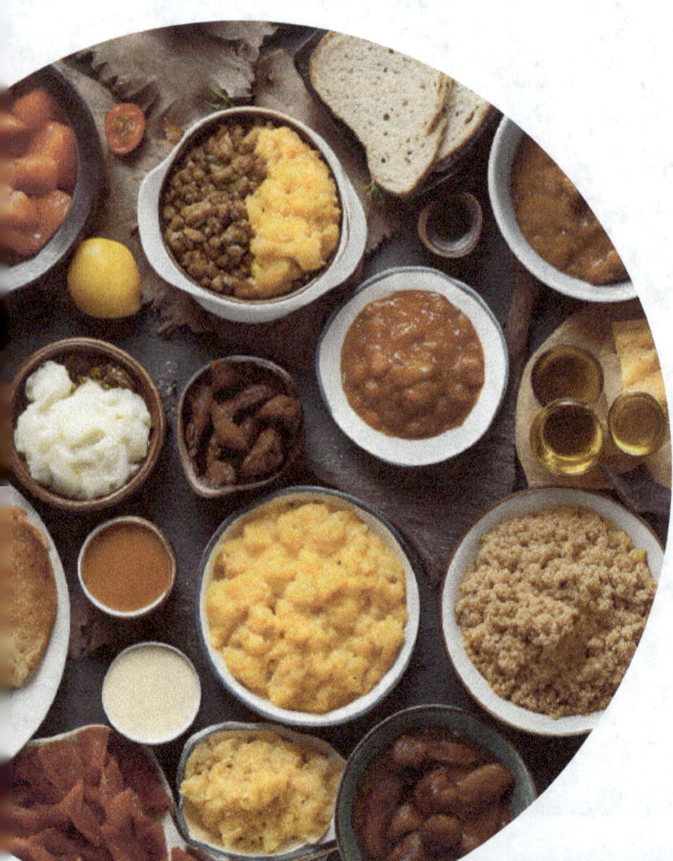

# Chapter 2: Understanding Diabetes

## What is Diabetes?

Diabetes is a chronic condition that affects how your body turns food into energy. Normally, when you eat, your body breaks down carbohydrates into glucose (sugar), which enters your bloodstream. The pancreas then releases insulin, a hormone that helps glucose enter your cells to be used for energy. In people with diabetes, this process is impaired, leading to high levels of glucose in the blood.

## Types of Diabetes

**1. Type 1 Diabetes:** An autoimmune condition where the body's immune system attacks the insulin-producing cells in the pancreas. People with Type 1 diabetes need to take insulin daily to manage their blood sugar levels.

**2. Type 2 Diabetes:** The most common form of diabetes, usually developing in adults, though increasingly seen in younger individuals due to lifestyle factors. It occurs when the body becomes resistant to insulin or when the pancreas doesn't produce enough insulin. Lifestyle changes and medication are often used to manage Type 2 diabetes.

**3. Gestational Diabetes:** This type of diabetes develops during pregnancy and usually goes away after the baby is born. However, it increases the risk of developing Type 2 diabetes later in life.

## The Role of Diet in Diabetes Management

Diet plays a crucial role in managing diabetes. The right food choices can help control blood sugar levels, maintain a healthy weight, and prevent complications. A well-balanced diet for diabetics includes a variety of nutrients and emphasizes portion control, nutrient-dense foods, and regular meal timing.

## Key Nutrients for Diabetics

1. Fiber: Found in fruits, vegetables, whole grains, and legumes, fiber helps slow down the absorption of sugar, preventing spikes in blood glucose levels.

2. Healthy Fats: Unsaturated fats from sources like nuts, seeds, avocados, and olive oil can improve heart health and provide essential nutrients.

3. Lean Protein: Protein from sources such as poultry, fish, beans, and tofu helps keep you full and supports muscle maintenance.

4. Complex Carbohydrates: Whole grains, starchy vegetables, and legumes provide sustained energy and are less likely to cause blood sugar spikes compared to refined carbohydrates.

## Tips for Reading Food Labels

1. Check Serving Sizes: Ensure that the serving size on the label matches the amount you plan to eat.

2. Look for Carbohydrate Content: Pay attention to the total carbohydrates, including fiber and sugars. Choose options with higher fiber content and lower added sugars.

3. Identify Healthy Fats: Opt for products with unsaturated fats and minimal saturated and trans fats.

4. Monitor Sodium Levels: Choose low-sodium options to help manage blood pressure and reduce the risk of heart disease.

## Planning Balanced Meals

Creating balanced meals can help manage diabetes effectively. Here's a simple guide to planning your meals:

1. Fill Half Your Plate with Non-Starchy Vegetables: Include a variety of colorful vegetables like leafy greens, broccoli, peppers, and tomatoes.

2. Include Lean Protein: Fill one-quarter of your plate with lean protein sources such as chicken, fish, tofu, or legumes.

3. Add Whole Grains or Starchy Vegetables: Use the remaining quarter for whole grains like quinoa, brown rice, or starchy vegetables like sweet potatoes.

4. Incorporate Healthy Fats: Add a small amount of healthy fats, such as a drizzle of olive oil, a handful of nuts, or slices of avocado.

5. Enjoy Fresh Fruits in Moderation: While fruits are nutritious, they contain natural sugars. Choose fruits with a lower glycemic index and watch portion sizes.

*By understanding the basics of diabetes and how diet impacts your health, you can make informed choices that support your well-being. The recipes in this cookbook are designed to help you enjoy the flavors of soul food while keeping your blood sugar levels in check. Together, we can embrace a lifestyle that celebrates tradition and promotes health.*

# Chapter 3 : Breakfast

## 1. English Sweet Potato Pancakes

- **Preparation Time:** 15 minutes
- **Cook Time:** 20 minutes
- **Total Time:** 35 minutes
- **Serves:** 4

### Ingredients

- 1 large sweet potato, peeled and grated
- 1 cup all-purpose flour
- 2 tbsp brown sugar
- 1 tsp baking powder
- 1/2 tsp ground cinnamon
- 1/4 tsp ground nutmeg
- 1/4 tsp salt
- 2 large eggs
- 1 cup milk
- 2 tbsp melted butter
- 1 tsp vanilla extract
- Butter or oil for cooking

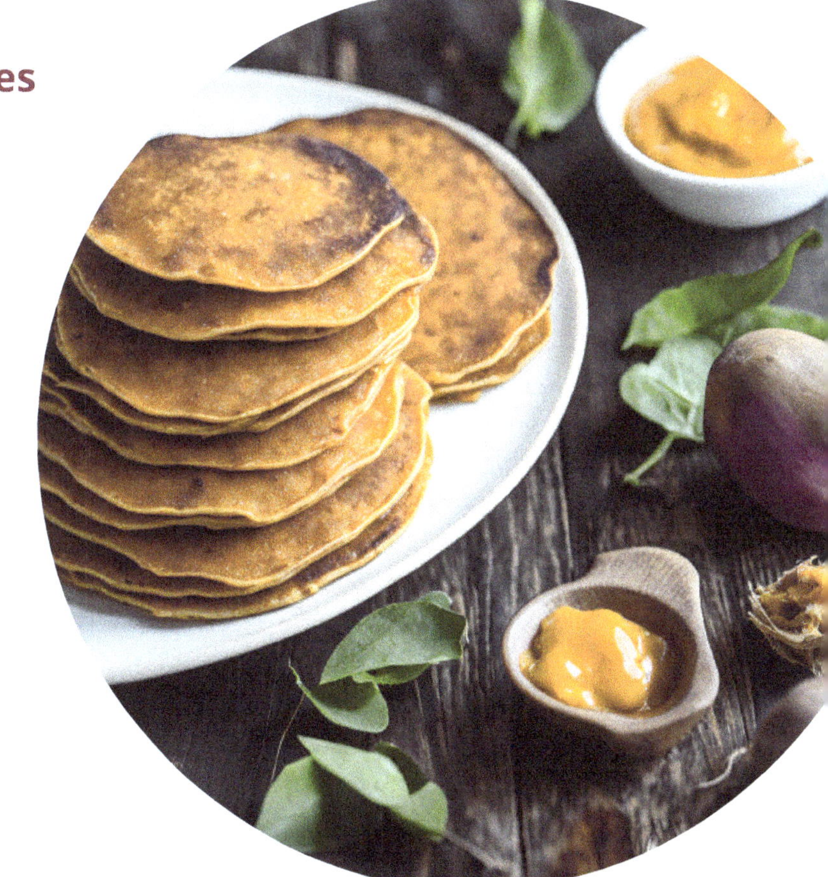

### Directions

1. In a large bowl, combine the grated sweet potato, flour, brown sugar, baking powder, cinnamon, nutmeg, and salt.

2. In a separate bowl, whisk together the eggs, milk, melted butter, and vanilla extract.

3. Pour the wet ingredients into the dry ingredients and stir until just combined. Do not overmix.

4. Heat a non-stick skillet or griddle over medium heat and add a little butter or oil.

5. Pour about 1/4 cup of batter onto the skillet for each pancake. Cook until bubbles form on the surface and the edges look set, about 2-3 minutes.

6. Flip the pancakes and cook for another 2-3 minutes, until golden brown and cooked through. Serve warm with your favorite toppings such as maple syrup, fresh fruit, or a dollop of yogurt.

### Nutrition Facts

Calories: 210 | Total Fat: 7g | Saturated Fat: 3g | Cholesterol: 95mg | Sodium: 220mg | Total Carbohydrates: 30g | Dietary Fiber: 2g | Sugar : 8g | Protein: 5g

# Chapter 3 : Breakfast

## 2. Spinach and Turkey Sausage Omelet

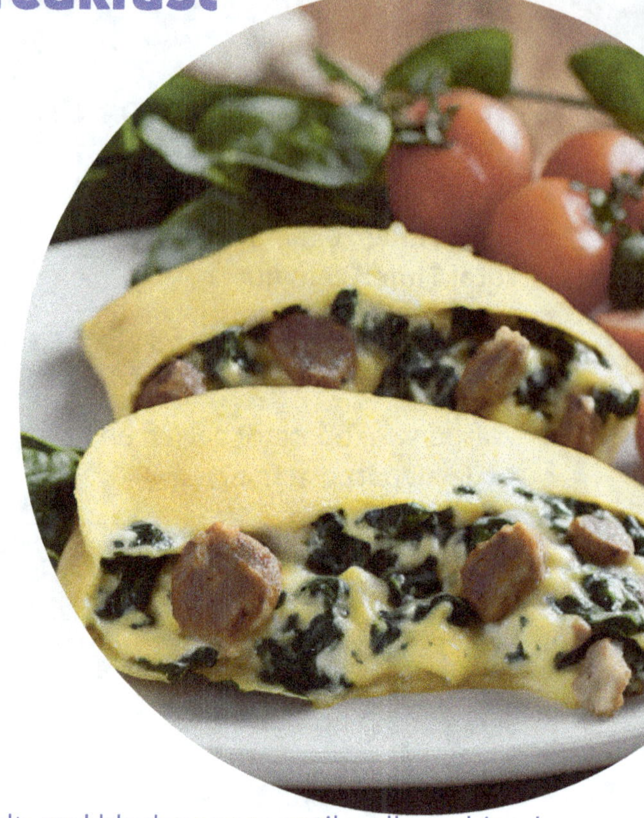

- **Preparation Time:** 10 minutes
- **Cook Time:** 10 minutes
- **Total Time:** 20 minutes
- **Serves:** 2

### Ingredients
- 4 large eggs
- 1/4 cup milk
- 1/4 tsp salt
- 1/4 tsp black pepper
- 1 tbsp olive oil
- 1/2 cup cooked turkey sausage, crumbled
- 1 cup fresh spinach, chopped
- 1/2 cup shredded cheddar cheese

### Directions
1. In a medium bowl, whisk together the eggs, milk, salt, and black pepper until well combined.
2. Heat the olive oil in a non-stick skillet over medium heat.

3. Add the turkey sausage and cook for 2-3 minutes, until warmed through.

4. Add the spinach and cook for another 1-2 minutes, until wilted.

5. Pour the egg mixture over the sausage and spinach. Cook without stirring until the eggs begin to set around the edges, about 2 minutes.

6. Using a spatula, gently lift the edges of the omelet and tilt the pan to allow the uncooked eggs to flow underneath.

7. Once the eggs are mostly set but still slightly runny on top, sprinkle the shredded cheddar cheese over half of the omelet.

8. Fold the omelet in half over the cheese and cook for another 1-2 minutes, until the cheese is melted and the eggs are fully set.

9. Slide the omelet onto a plate and serve immediately.

### Nutrition Facts
Calories: 310 | Total Fat: 22g | Saturated Fat: 8g | Cholesterol: 345mg | Sodium: 720mg | Total Carbohydrates: 3g | Dietary Fiber: 1g | Sugar: 1g | Protein: 24g

# Chapter 3 : Breakfast

### 3. Southern Grits with a Twist

- **Preparation Time:** 10 minutes
- **Cook Time:** 20 minutes
- **Total Time:** 30 minutes
- **Serves**: 4

## Ingredients

- 1 cup stone-ground grits
- 4 cups water
- 1 cup shredded sharp cheddar cheese
- 1/2 cup cooked and crumbled bacon
- 1/2 cup diced green onions
- 1/4 cup heavy cream
- 2 tbsp butter
- 1/2 tsp salt
- 1/4 tsp black pepper

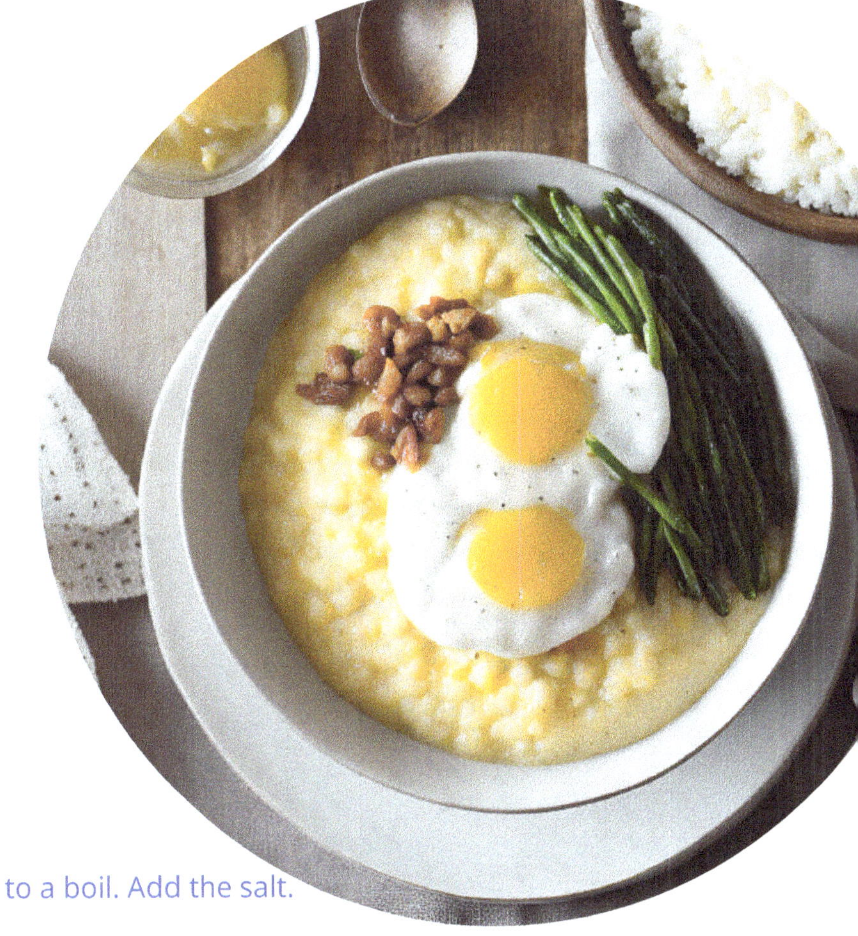

### Directions

1. In a medium saucepan, bring the water to a boil. Add the salt.

2. Slowly stir in the grits and reduce the heat to low. Cook, stirring frequently, for about 15-20 minutes, or until the grits are thick and creamy.

3. Remove the saucepan from heat and stir in the butter, heavy cream, shredded cheddar cheese, cooked bacon, and diced green onions.

4. Season with black pepper and additional salt to taste if needed.

5. Serve hot, garnished with extra cheese, bacon, and green onions if desired.

## Nutrition Facts

Calories: 350 | Total Fat: 22g | Saturated Fat: 12g | Cholesterol: 70mg | Sodium: 810mg | Total Carbohydrates: 26g | Dietary Fiber: 1g | Sugar: 0g | Protein: 10g

## 4. Low-Sugar Peach Cobbler Smoothie

- Preparation Time: 5 minutes
- Cook Time: 0 minutes
- Total Time: 5 minutes
- Serves: 2

### Ingredients

- 2 cups frozen peaches
- 1 cup unsweetened almond milk
- 1/2 cup plain Greek yogurt
- 1/4 cup rolled oats
- 1/2 tsp ground cinnamon
- 1/4 tsp ground nutmeg
- 1 tsp vanilla extract
- 1 tbsp chia seeds
- Ice cubes (optional)

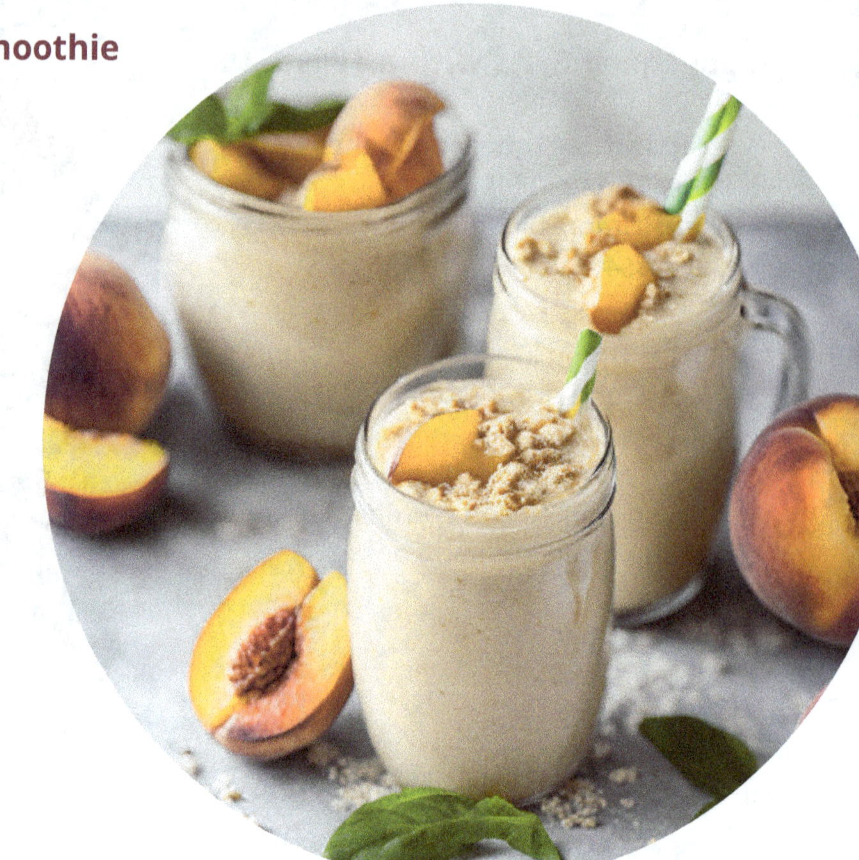

### Directions

1. In a blender, combine the frozen peaches, almond milk, Greek yogurt, rolled oats, ground cinnamon, ground nutmeg, vanilla extract, and chia seeds.

2. Blend on high until smooth and creamy. If the smoothie is too thick, add more almond milk or a few ice cubes and blend again.

3. Pour into glasses and serve immediately.

### Nutrition Facts

Calories: 180 | Total Fat: 5g | Saturated Fat: 1g | Cholesterol: 5mg | Sodium: 60mg | Total Carbohydrates: 28g | Dietary Fiber: 5g | Sugar: 12g | Protein: 8g

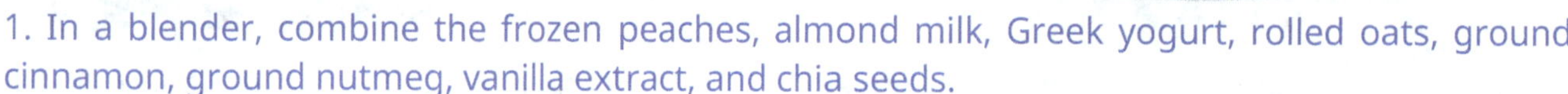

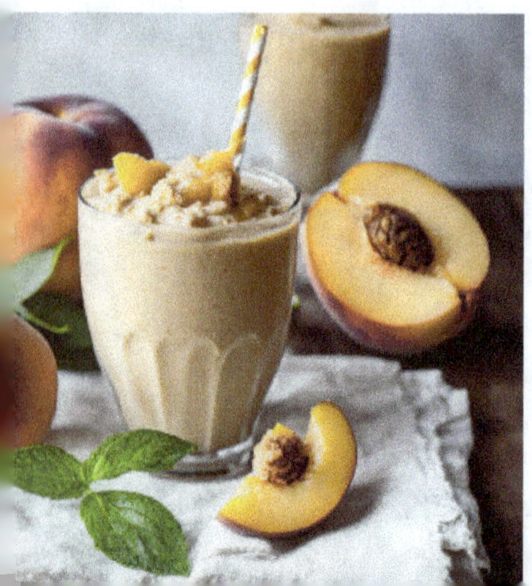
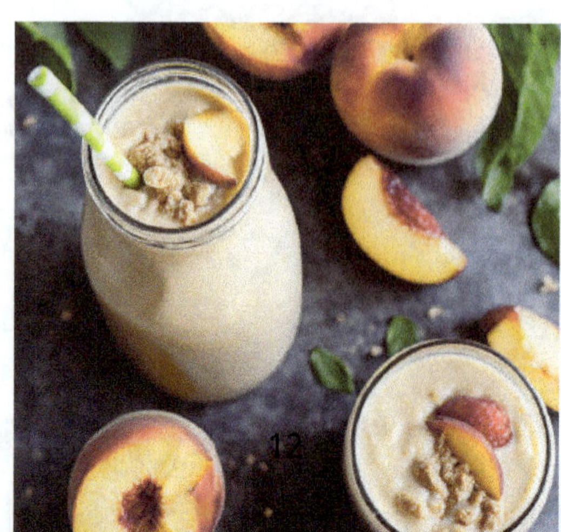
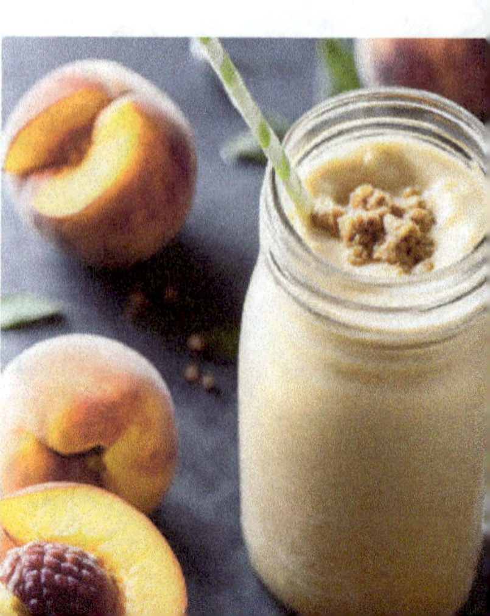

## 5. Veggie-Stuffed Breakfast Burrito

- **Preparation Time: 1**0 minutes
- **Cook Time:** 15 minutes
- **Total Time:** 25 minutes
- **Serves:** 4

## Ingredients

- 4 large whole wheat tortillas
- 6 large eggs
- 1/4 cup milk
- 1 tbsp olive oil
- 1 cup diced bell peppers (any color)
- 1/2 cup diced onions
- 1 cup baby spinach, chopped
- 1/2 cup shredded cheddar cheese
- 1/4 cup salsa
- 1 avocado, sliced
- Salt and pepper to taste

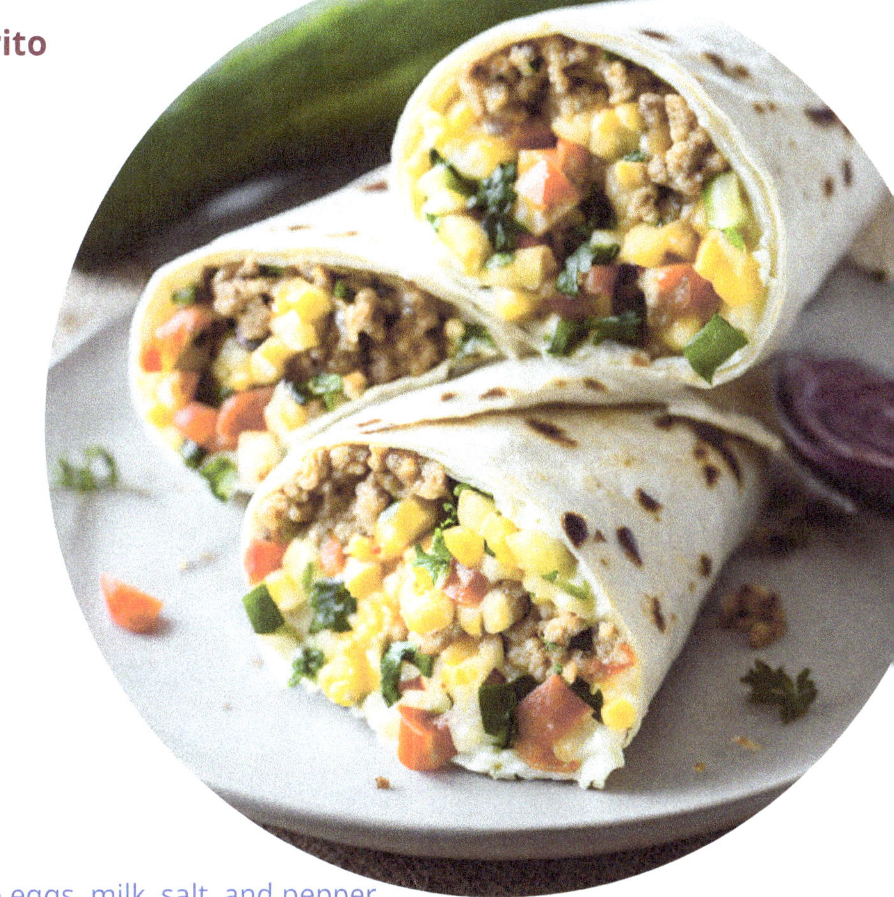

## Directions

1. In a medium bowl, whisk together the eggs, milk, salt, and pepper.

2. Heat the olive oil in a large non-stick skillet over medium heat.

3. Add the diced bell peppers and onions to the skillet. Cook for 5-7 minutes, until softened.

4. Add the chopped spinach to the skillet and cook for another 2 minutes, until wilted.

5. Pour the egg mixture into the skillet. Cook, stirring occasionally, until the eggs are scrambled and fully cooked, about 5 minutes.

6. Remove the skillet from heat and stir in the shredded cheddar cheese until melted.

7. Warm the tortillas in the microwave or on a skillet for about 20 seconds each.

8. Divide the scrambled egg mixture evenly among the tortillas. Top with salsa and sliced avocado. Roll up the tortillas, folding in the sides to form burritos. Serve immediately.

## Nutrition Facts

Calories: 320 | Total Fat: 18g | Saturated Fat: 6g | Cholesterol: 250mg | Sodium: 520mg | Total Carbohydrates: 26g | Dietary Fiber: 6g | Sugar: 3g | Protein: 16g

## 6. Cinnamon Oatmeal with Berries

- **Preparation Time:** 5 minutes
- **Cook Time:** 10 minutes
- **Total Time:** 15 minutes
- **Serves:** 2

## Ingredients

- 1 cup rolled oats
- 2 cups water or milk
- 1/2 tsp ground cinnamon
- 1/4 tsp salt
- 1 tbsp honey or maple syrup
- 1/2 cup mixed berries
(strawberries, blueberries, raspberries)
- 2 tbsp chopped nuts (optional)
- 1/2 tsp vanilla extract (optional)

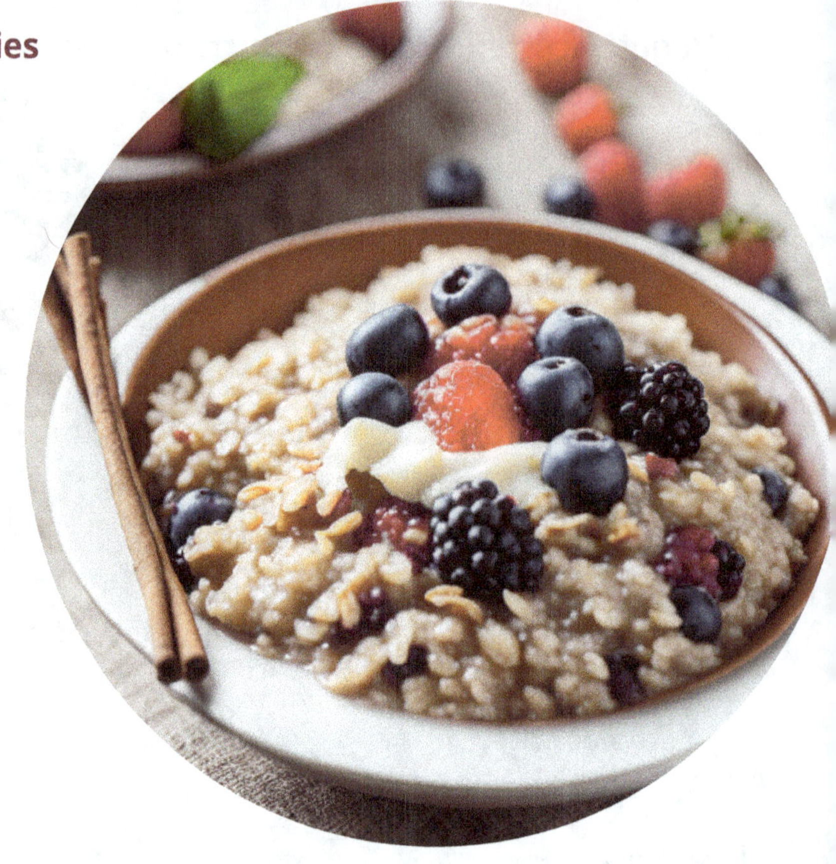

## Directions

1. In a medium saucepan, bring the water or milk to a boil. Add the salt.

2. Stir in the rolled oats and reduce the heat to low. Cook, stirring occasionally, for about 5 minutes or until the oats are tender and have absorbed most of the liquid.

3. Stir in the ground cinnamon, honey or maple syrup, and vanilla extract if using.

4. Remove the saucepan from heat and let the oatmeal sit for a minute to thicken.

5. Divide the oatmeal into two bowls. Top with mixed berries and chopped nuts if desired.

6. Serve hot and enjoy!

**Nutrition Facts**

Calories: 220 | Total Fat: 6g | Saturated Fat: 1g | Cholesterol: 0mg | Sodium: 150mg | Total Carbohydrates: 38g | Dietary Fiber: 6g | Sugar: 12g | Protein: 6g

# Chapter 3 : Breakfast

## 7. Collard Green and Mushroom Frittata

- **Preparation Time:** 10 minutes
- **Cook Time:** 20 minutes
- **Total Time:** 30 minutes
- **Serves:** 4

## Ingredients

- 8 large eggs
- 1/4 cup milk or heavy cream
- 1/2 tsp salt
- 1/4 tsp black pepper
- 1 tbsp olive oil
- 1 cup chopped collard greens, tough stems removed
- 1 cup sliced mushrooms (such as cremini or button mushrooms)
- 1/2 cup diced onion
- 1 garlic clove, minced
- 1/2 cup shredded mozzarella cheese
- 1/4 cup grated Parmesan cheese
- Fresh parsley or chives for garnish (optional)

## Directions

1. Preheat your oven to 350°F (175°C).

2. In a large bowl, whisk together the eggs, milk or heavy cream, salt, and black pepper until well combined. Set aside.

3. Heat the olive oil in an oven-safe skillet over medium heat.

4. Add the chopped collard greens, sliced mushrooms, diced onion, and minced garlic to the skillet. Cook, stirring occasionally, for about 5 minutes or until the vegetables are softened.

5. Pour the egg mixture evenly over the vegetables in the skillet. Stir gently to distribute the vegetables throughout the eggs.

6. Sprinkle the shredded mozzarella and grated Parmesan cheese evenly over the top of the frittata.

7. Transfer the skillet to the preheated oven and bake for 15-18 minutes, or until the eggs are set and the cheese is melted and lightly browned.

8. Remove the frittata from the oven and let it cool slightly before slicing.

9. Garnish with fresh parsley or chives if desired. Serve warm.

## Nutrition Facts

Calories: 250 | Total Fat: 16g | Saturated Fat: 6g | Cholesterol: 380mg | Sodium: 540mg | Total Carbohydrates: 7g | Dietary Fiber: 2g | Sugar: 2g | Protein: 19g

# Chapter 4 : Lunch

## Grilled Chicken and Kale Salad

- **Preparation Time:** 15 minutes
- **Cook Time:** 15 minutes
- **Total Time:** 30 minutes
- **Serves:** 2

### Ingredients

- 2 boneless, skinless chicken breasts
- Salt and pepper to taste
- 1 tbsp olive oil
- 4 cups chopped kale leaves, tough stems removed
- 1 cup cherry tomatoes, halved
- 1/2 cup cucumber, sliced
- 1/4 cup red onion, thinly sliced
- 1/4 cup crumbled feta cheese
- 2 tbsp sunflower seeds (optional)
- Lemon wedges for serving

*For the Dressing:*
- 3 tbsp olive oil
- 2 tbsp lemon juice
- 1 tsp Dijon mustard
- 1 clove garlic, minced
- Salt and pepper to taste

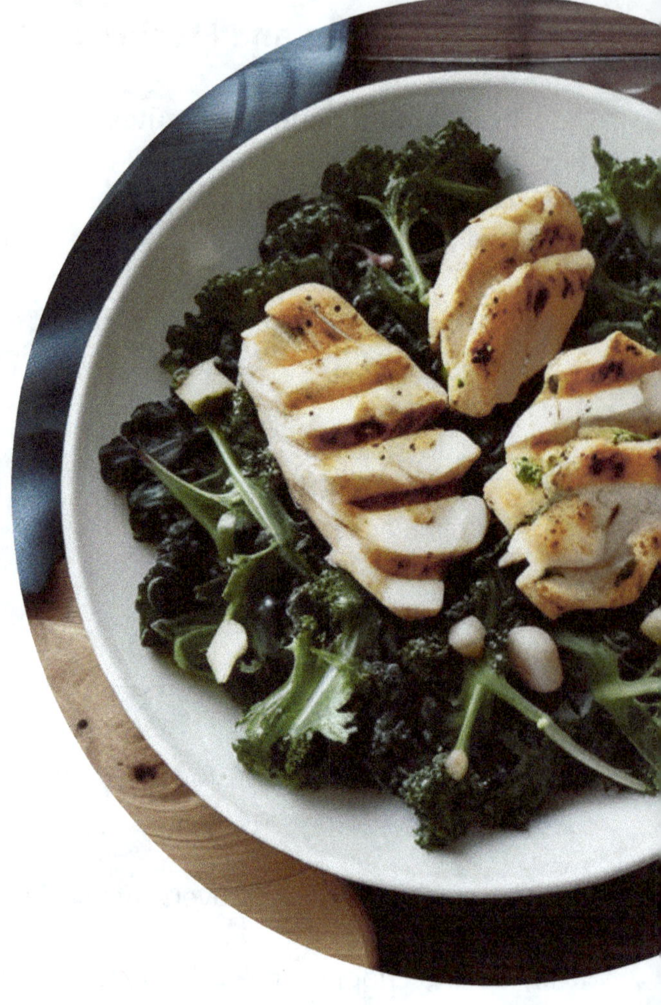

### Directions

1. Preheat a grill or grill pan over medium-high heat.
2. Season the chicken breasts with salt, pepper, and olive oil. Grill the chicken for about 6-7 minutes per side, or until cooked through and no longer pink in the center. Remove from heat and let it rest for a few minutes before slicing.
3. In a large bowl, combine the chopped kale, cherry tomatoes, cucumber, and red onion.
4. In a small bowl or jar, whisk together the olive oil, lemon juice, Dijon mustard, minced garlic, salt, and pepper to make the dressing.
5. Pour the dressing over the kale salad and toss to coat evenly.
6. Divide the dressed salad between two plates. Top each with sliced grilled chicken.
7. Sprinkle crumbled feta cheese and sunflower seeds over the salads.
8. Serve with lemon wedges on the side for squeezing over the salad before eating.

### Nutrition Facts

Calories: 450 | Total Fat: 28g | Saturated Fat: 6g | Cholesterol: 90mg | Sodium: 380mg | Total Carbohydrates: 20g | Dietary Fiber: 4g | Sugar: 5g | Protein: 32g

## Black-Eyed Pea Soup

- **Preparation Time:** 10 minutes
- **Cook Time:** 1 hour 15 minutes
- **Total Time:** 1 hour 25 minutes
- **Serves:** 6

## Ingredients

- 1 cup dried black-eyed peas, rinsed and drained
- 1 tbsp olive oil
- 1 onion, chopped
- 2 carrots, peeled and diced
- 2 celery stalks, diced
- 3 cloves garlic, minced
- 6 cups vegetable or chicken broth
- 1 bay leaf
- 1 tsp dried thyme
- 1/2 tsp smoked paprika
- Salt and pepper to taste
- Chopped fresh parsley for garnish (optional)

## Directions

1. In a large pot, heat the olive oil over medium heat. Add the chopped onion, carrots, and celery. Cook, stirring occasionally, for about 5 minutes or until the vegetables begin to soften.

2. Add the minced garlic to the pot and cook for another minute until fragrant.

3. Stir in the dried black-eyed peas, vegetable or chicken broth, bay leaf, dried thyme, and smoked paprika. Bring the mixture to a boil.

4. Reduce the heat to low, cover the pot, and simmer for 1 hour or until the black-eyed peas are tender.

5. Remove the bay leaf from the soup. Taste and adjust seasoning with salt and pepper as needed.

6. If desired, use an immersion blender to partially blend the soup for a creamier texture, leaving some peas whole. Ladle the soup into bowls and garnish with chopped fresh parsley, if desired. Serve hot with crusty bread or a side salad.

## Nutrition Facts

Calories: 200 | Total Fat: 4g | Saturated Fat: 0.5g | Cholesterol: 0mg | Sodium: 800mg | Total Carbohydrates: 34g | Dietary Fiber: 8g | Sugar: 6g | Protein: 9g

## Spicy Shrimp and Avocado Wrap

- **Preparation Time:** 15 minutes
- **Cook Time:** 10 minutes
- **Total Time:** 25 minutes
- **Serves:** 2

## Ingredients

- 8 large shrimp, peeled and deveined
- 1 tbsp olive oil
- 1/2 tsp paprika
- 1/4 tsp cayenne pepper (adjust to taste)
- Salt and pepper to taste
- 2 large whole wheat tortillas
- 1/2 avocado, sliced
- 1/2 cup shredded lettuce
- 1/4 cup diced tomatoes
- 1/4 cup diced red onion
- 1/4 cup plain Greek yogurt or sour cream
- Fresh cilantro leaves for garnish (optional)
- Lime wedges for serving

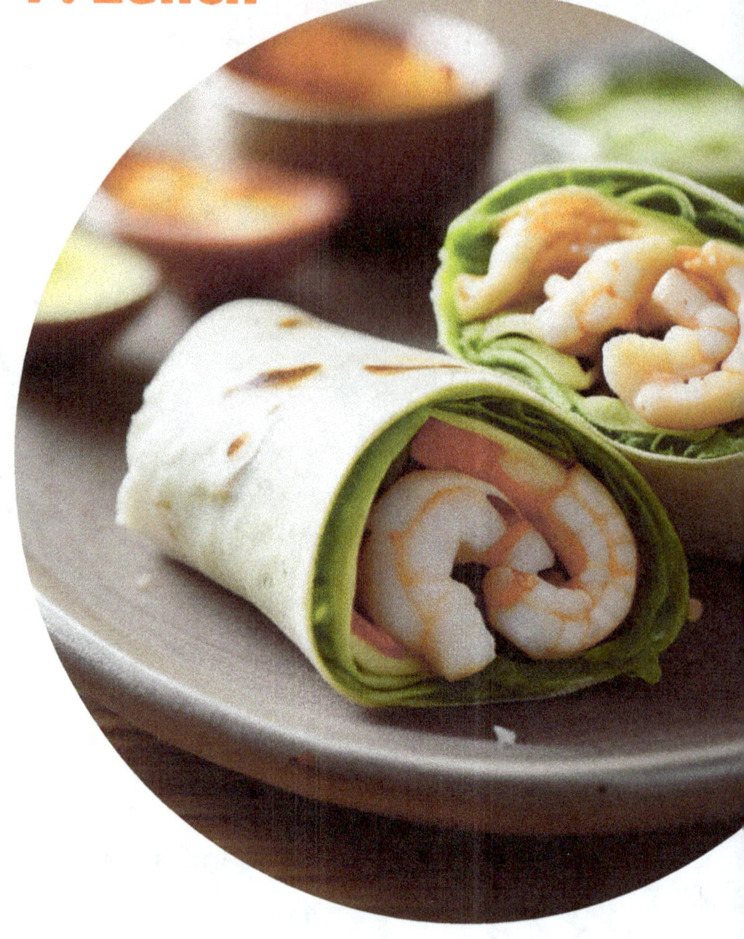

## Directions

1. In a bowl, toss the shrimp with olive oil, paprika, cayenne pepper, salt, and pepper until evenly coated.
2. Heat a skillet over medium-high heat. Add the seasoned shrimp and cook for 2-3 minutes per side, or until the shrimp are pink and cooked through.
3. Remove the shrimp from the skillet and set aside.
4. Warm the whole wheat tortillas in the skillet for about 20 seconds on each side, or until they are pliable.
5. To assemble the wraps, spread a layer of Greek yogurt or sour cream on each tortilla.
6. Divide the shredded lettuce, diced tomatoes, diced red onion, sliced avocado, and cooked shrimp evenly between the tortillas.
7. Garnish with fresh cilantro leaves if desired.
8. Squeeze fresh lime juice over the fillings.
9. Roll up the tortillas, folding in the sides to secure the fillings.
10. Cut each wrap in half diagonally and serve immediately.

## Nutrition Facts

Calories: 350 | Total Fat: 16g | Saturated Fat: 3g | Cholesterol: 95mg | Sodium: 520mg | Total Carbohydrates: 34g | Dietary Fiber: 7g | Sugar: 3g | Protein: 20g

## Turkey and Collard Green Sandwich

- **Preparation Time:** 10 minutes
- **Cook Time:** 5 minutes
- **Total Time:** 15 minutes
- **Serves:** 2

## Ingredients

- 4 slices whole grain bread
- 1/2 lb thinly sliced turkey breast
- 1 cup cooked collard greens (leftover or prepared)
- 1/2 cup sliced tomatoes
- 1/4 cup thinly sliced red onion
- 2 tbsp mayonnaise or mustard (optional)
- Salt and pepper to taste

## Directions

1. Toast the slices of whole grain bread until lightly golden and crispy.

2. If desired, spread mayonnaise or mustard on one side of each slice of bread.

3. Layer the thinly sliced turkey breast on two slices of bread.

4. Top the turkey with cooked collard greens, sliced tomatoes, and thinly sliced red onion.

5. Season with salt and pepper to taste.

6. Place the remaining slices of bread on top to form sandwiches.

7. Cut the sandwiches in half diagonally and serve immediately.

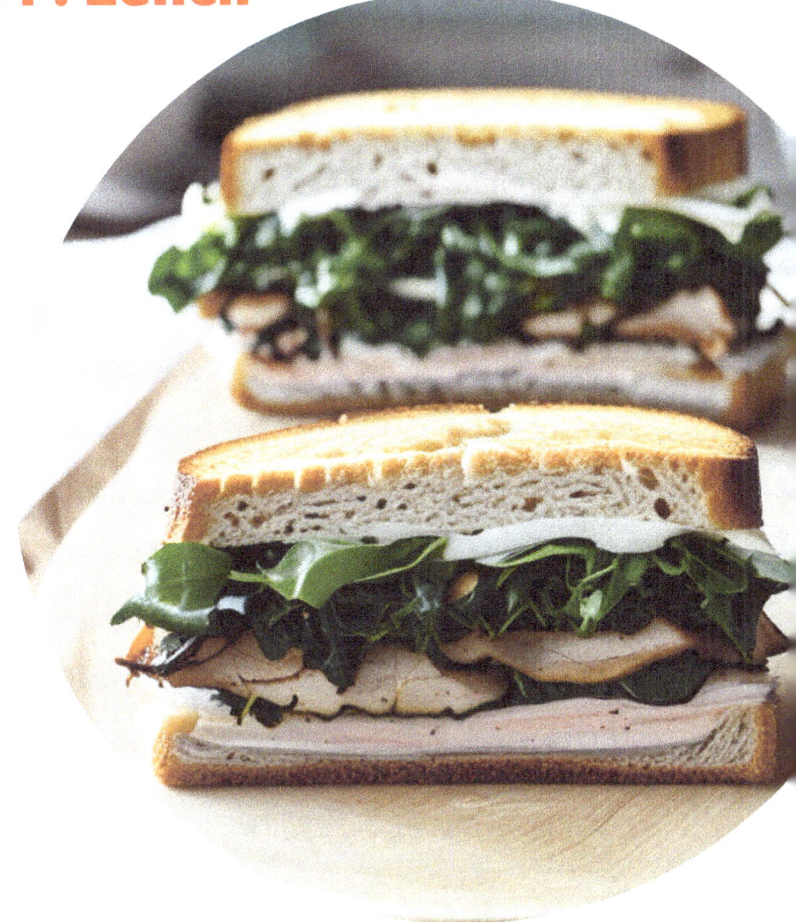

## Quinoa and Black Bean Bowl

- **Preparation Time:** 10 minutes
- **Cook Time:** 20 minutes
- **Total Time:** 30 minutes
- **Serves:** 2

### Ingredients

- 1/2 cup quinoa, rinsed
- 1 cup water or vegetable broth
- 1 cup canned black beans, rinsed and drained
- 1 cup corn kernels (fresh or frozen)
- 1 cup cherry tomatoes, halved
- 1/2 avocado, diced
- 1/4 cup chopped fresh cilantro
- 2 tbsp lime juice
- 1 tbsp olive oil
- 1/2 tsp ground cumin
- Salt and pepper to taste
- Optional toppings: diced red onion, sliced jalapeños, crumbled feta cheese

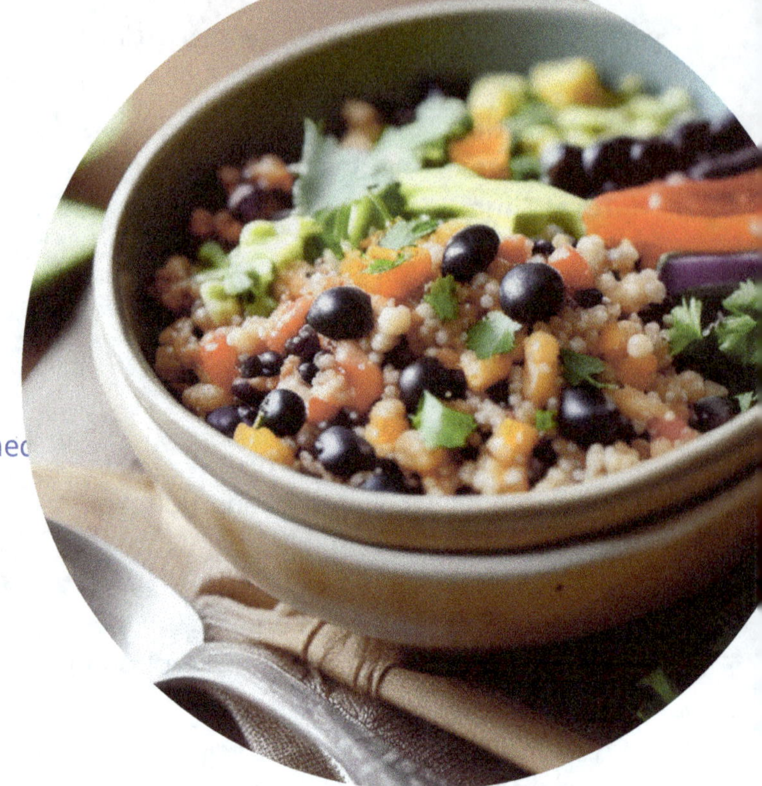

## Directions

1. In a medium saucepan, combine the quinoa and water or vegetable broth. Bring to a boil over medium-high heat.

2. Reduce the heat to low, cover, and simmer for about 15-20 minutes, or until the quinoa is cooked and the liquid is absorbed. Remove from heat and let it sit, covered, for 5 minutes.

3. Fluff the quinoa with a fork and let it cool slightly.

4. In a large bowl, combine the cooked quinoa, black beans, corn kernels, cherry tomatoes, diced avocado, and chopped fresh cilantro.

5. In a small bowl, whisk together the lime juice, olive oil, ground cumin, salt, and pepper.

6. Pour the dressing over the quinoa mixture and toss gently to combine.

7. Divide the quinoa and black bean mixture into bowls.

8. Garnish with optional toppings like diced red onion, sliced jalapeños, or crumbled feta cheese if desired. Serve immediately and enjoy

# Chapter 4 : Lunch

## Southern-Style Stuffed Bell Peppers

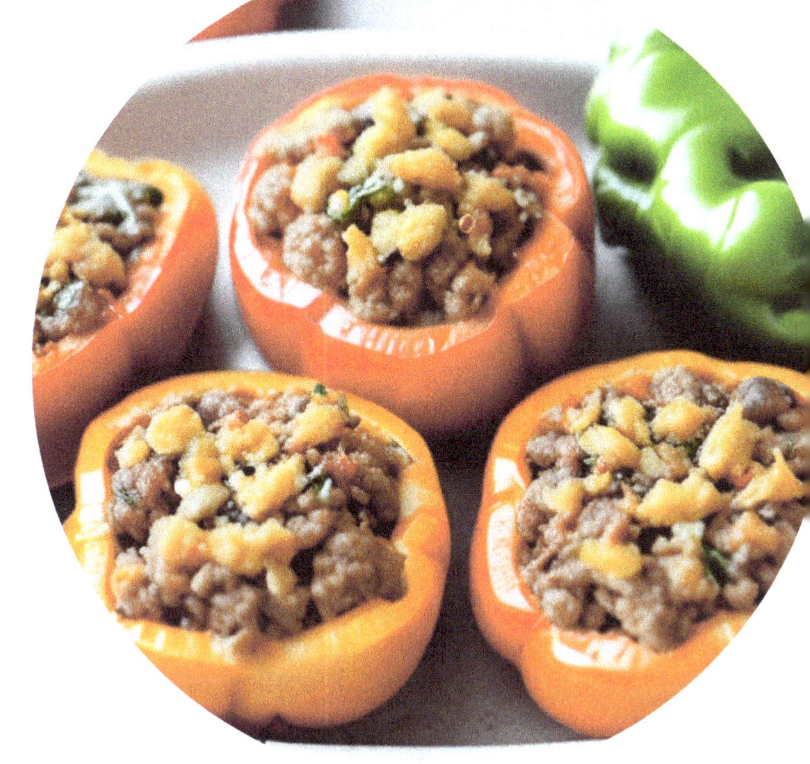

- **Preparation Time:** 20 minutes
- **Cook Time:** 1 hour
- **Total Time:** 1 hour 20 minutes
- **Serves:** 4

### Ingredients

- 4 large bell peppers (any color), tops cut off and seeds removed
- 1 lb ground beef or turkey
- 1 cup cooked rice (white or brown)
- 1/2 cup diced onion
- 1/2 cup diced celery
- 1/2 cup diced bell pepper (from tops)
- 2 cloves garlic, minced
- 1 can (14 oz) diced tomatoes, drained
- 1 cup shredded cheddar cheese
- 1 tsp dried oregano
- 1 tsp dried thyme
- 1/2 tsp smoked paprika
- Salt and pepper to taste
- Chopped fresh parsley for garnish

### Directions

1. Preheat your oven to 375°F (190°C).
2. Bring a large pot of water to a boil. Add the bell peppers and cook for 3-4 minutes, until slightly softened. Remove from water and set aside to cool.
3. In a large skillet, cook the ground beef or turkey over medium heat until browned and cooked through. Drain any excess fat.
4. Add the diced onion, celery, diced bell pepper, and minced garlic to the skillet. Cook for 5 minutes, until vegetables are softened.
5. Stir in the cooked rice, drained diced tomatoes, dried oregano, dried thyme, smoked paprika, salt, and pepper. Cook for another 2-3 minutes, until heated through.
6. Remove the skillet from heat and stir in half of the shredded cheddar cheese.
7. Stuff each bell pepper with the meat and rice mixture, packing it tightly.
8. Place the stuffed bell peppers upright in a baking dish. If there is leftover filling, spoon it around the peppers in the dish.
9. Cover the baking dish with foil and bake in the preheated oven for 30 minutes.
10. Remove the foil, sprinkle the remaining shredded cheddar cheese over the tops of the peppers, and bake uncovered for another 10-15 minutes, until cheese is melted and bubbly.
11. Remove from oven and let the peppers cool slightly before serving.
12. Garnish with chopped fresh parsley before serving

# Chapter 4 : Lunch

**Catfish Tacos with Mango Salsa**

- **Preparation Time:** 20 minutes
- **Cook Time:** 15 minutes
- **Total Time:** 35 minutes
- **Serves:** 4

**Ingredients**

## For the Catfish Tacos:
- 1 lb catfish fillets, cut into strips
- 1 tbsp olive oil
- 1 tsp ground cumin
- 1/2 tsp chili powder
- Salt and pepper to taste
- 8 small corn or flour tortillas
- Shredded cabbage or lettuce, for serving
- Lime wedges, for serving

## For the Mango Salsa:
- 1 ripe mango, peeled and diced
- 1/2 cup diced red bell pepper
- 1/4 cup diced red onion
- 1/4 cup chopped fresh cilantro
- Juice of 1 lime
- Salt and pepper to taste

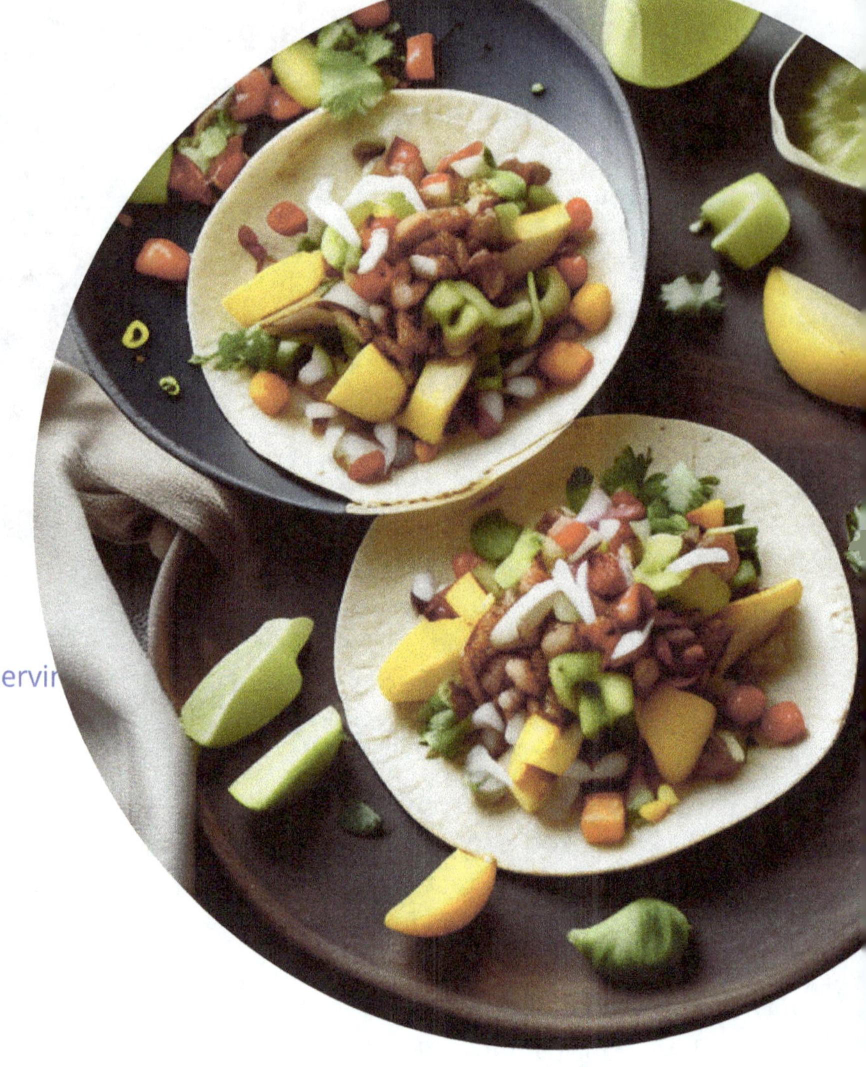

## Directions

1. In a bowl, combine the olive oil, ground cumin, chili powder, salt, and pepper. Add the catfish strips and toss to coat evenly.

2. Heat a skillet over medium-high heat. Add the catfish strips and cook for 3-4 minutes per side, or until the fish is cooked through and flakes easily with a fork. Remove from heat and set aside.

3. In a separate bowl, combine all the ingredients for the mango salsa: diced mango, diced red bell pepper, diced red onion, chopped fresh cilantro, lime juice, salt, and pepper. Mix well.

4. Warm the tortillas in a dry skillet or microwave until soft and pliable.

5. To assemble the tacos, place some shredded cabbage or lettuce on each tortilla. Top with catfish strips and spoonfuls of mango salsa.

6. Serve the catfish tacos with lime wedges on the side for squeezing over the tacos. Enjoy your delicious Catfish Tacos with Mango Salsa

# Chapter 5 : Dinner

## Baked BBQ Chicken with Steamed Vegetables

**Preparation Time:** 15 minutes | Cook Time: 45 minutes | Total Time: 1 hour | Serves: 4

### Ingredients:

Chicken Breasts, Barbecue Sauce, Olive Oil, Salt, Pepper, Broccoli, Carrots, Zucchini

### Directions:

1. Preheat oven to 400°F.

2. Season chicken breasts with salt and pepper.

3. Place chicken in a baking dish and brush with barbecue sauce.

4. Bake for 30-35 minutes, or until chicken is cooked through.

5. In a steamer basket, steam the broccoli, carrots, and zucchini for 10-12 minutes, or until tender.

6. Serve the baked BBQ chicken with the steamed vegetables.

### Nutrition Facts:

Calories: 420 | Total Fat: 14g | Saturated Fat: 2g | Cholesterol: 186mg | Sodium: 1513mg | Total Carbohydrates: 49g | Dietary Fiber: 5g | Sugar: 6g | Protein: 24g

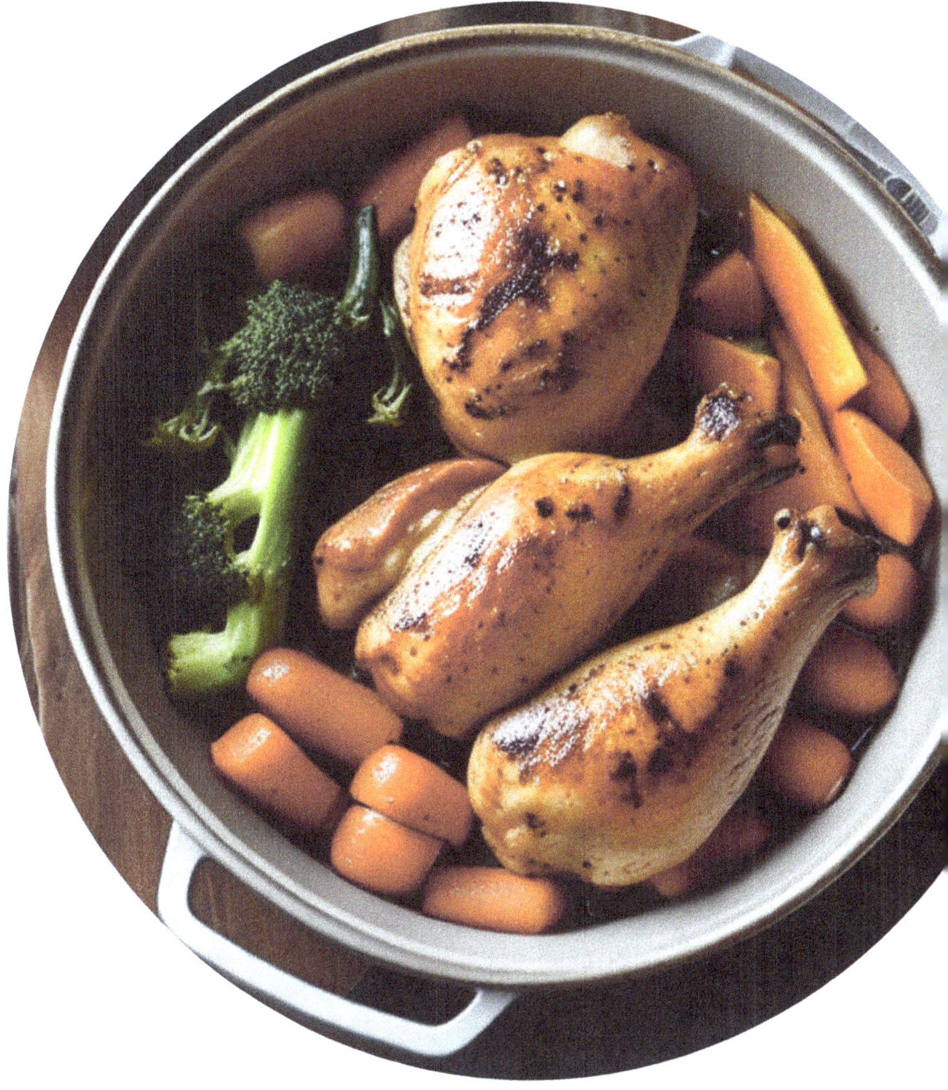

## Recipe: Low-Sodium Gumbo

Preparation Time: 30 minutes
Cook Time: 1 hour 30 minutes
Total Time: 2 hours
Serves: 6-8

### Ingredients:

- 1/4 cup olive oil
- 1/4 cup all-purpose flour
- 1 large onion, diced
- 1 green bell pepper, diced
- 3 celery stalks, diced
- 4 garlic cloves, minced
- 1 lb boneless, skinless chicken breasts, cut into 1-inch pieces
- 1 lb andouille sausage, sliced
- 4 cups low-sodium chicken broth
- 1 (14.5 oz) can diced tomatoes, no salt added
- 1 tsp dried thyme
- 1 tsp dried oregano
- 1/2 tsp cayenne pepper
- 1/4 tsp black pepper
- 2 bay leaves
- 1 lb peeled and deveined shrimp
- 1/4 cup chopped fresh parsley
- Cooked brown rice, for serving

**Nutrition Facts (per serving):**
Calories: 350
Total Fat: 16g
Saturated Fat: 4g
Cholesterol: 150mg
Sodium: 450mg
Total Carbohydrates: 20g
Fiber: 3g
Sugars: 4g
Protein: 32g

### Directions:

1. In a large pot or Dutch oven, heat the olive oil over medium heat. Whisk in the flour and cook, stirring constantly, for 10-15 minutes until the roux is a deep golden brown color.
2. Add the onion, bell pepper, celery, and garlic to the pot. Cook, stirring occasionally, for 5-7 minutes until the vegetables are softened.
3. Add the chicken and sausage to the pot. Cook for 5-7 minutes, stirring occasionally, until the chicken is lightly browned.
4. Pour in the chicken broth and add the diced tomatoes, thyme, oregano, cayenne, black pepper, and bay leaves. Bring the mixture to a boil, then reduce the heat and simmer for 45-60 minutes, stirring occasionally, until the flavors have melded.
5. Add the shrimp to the pot and cook for 5-7 minutes until the shrimp are opaque and cooked through.
6. Remove the bay leaves. Stir in the chopped parsley.
7. Serve the gumbo over cooked brown rice.

# Chapter 5 : Dinner

**Smothered Pork Chops with Cauliflower Mash**

Preparation Time: 20 minutes
Cook Time: 45 minutes
Total Time: 1 hour 5 minutes
Serves: 4

**Ingredients**:
***Pork Chops:***
- 4 bone-in pork chops (about 1-inch thick)
- 1 tbsp olive oil
- 1 onion, sliced
- 2 cloves garlic, minced
- 1 cup low-sodium chicken broth
- 1 tsp dried thyme
- 1/4 tsp black pepper

***Cauliflower Mash:***
- 1 head cauliflower, cut into florets
- 2 tbsp unsweetened almond milk
- 2 tbsp grated Parmesan cheese
- 1/4 tsp garlic powder
- 1/4 tsp salt
- 1/8 tsp black pepper

**Nutrition Facts (per serving):**
Calories: 350
Total Fat: 16g
Saturated Fat: 5g
Cholesterol: 90mg
Sodium: 450mg
Total Carbohydrates: 14g
Fiber: 4g
Sugars: 5g
Protein: 38g

**Directions:**
***Pork Chops:***
1. Season the pork chops with salt and pepper.
2. Heat the olive oil in a large skillet over medium-high heat. Add the pork chops and cook for 3-4 minutes per side until browned.
3. Remove the pork chops from the skillet and set aside.
4. Add the onion to the skillet and cook for 5 minutes, stirring occasionally, until softened.
5. Add the garlic and cook for 1 minute until fragrant.
6. Pour in the chicken broth and add the thyme and black pepper. Bring the mixture to a simmer.
7. Return the pork chops to the skillet, cover, and reduce heat to medium-low. Simmer for 25-30 minutes, turning the chops occasionally, until the pork is cooked through and tender.

**Cauliflower Mash:**
1. In a large pot, bring 1 inch of water to a boil. Add the cauliflower florets, cover, and steam for 10-12 minutes until very tender.
2. Drain the cauliflower and transfer to a food processor. Add the almond milk, Parmesan, garlic powder, salt, and black pepper.
3. Pulse the mixture until smooth and creamy.

# Chapter 5 : Dinner

**Jambalaya with Brown Rice**

Preparation Time: 20 minutes
Cook Time: 45 minutes
Total Time: 1 hour 5 minutes
Serves: 6

**Ingredients:**
- 1 cup uncooked brown rice
- 1 tbsp olive oil
- 1 lb boneless, skinless chicken breasts, cut into 1-inch pieces
- 1 lb andouille sausage, sliced
- 1 onion, diced
- 1 green bell pepper, diced
- 3 celery stalks, diced
- 3 garlic cloves, minced
- 1 (14.5 oz) can diced tomatoes, no salt added
- 2 cups low-sodium chicken broth
- 1 tsp dried thyme
- 1 tsp dried oregano
- 1/2 tsp cayenne pepper
- 1/4 tsp black pepper
- 1 bay leaf
- 1 lb peeled and deveined shrimp
- 2 tbsp chopped fresh parsley

**Nutrition Facts (per serving):**
Calories: 400
Total Fat: 14g
Saturated Fat: 4g
Cholesterol: 150mg
Sodium: 650mg
Total Carbohydrates: 35g
Fiber: 5g
Sugars: 5g
Protein: 35g

**Directions:**
1. Cook the brown rice according to package instructions. Set aside.

2. In a large pot or Dutch oven, heat the olive oil over medium-high heat. Add the chicken and sausage and cook for 5-7 minutes, stirring occasionally, until lightly browned.

3. Add the onion, bell pepper, celery, and garlic to the pot. Cook for 5-7 minutes, stirring occasionally, until the vegetables are softened.

4. Stir in the diced tomatoes, chicken broth, thyme, oregano, cayenne, black pepper, and bay leaf. Bring the mixture to a boil, then reduce the heat and simmer for 20-25 minutes.

5. Add the shrimp to the pot and cook for 5-7 minutes until the shrimp are opaque and cooked through.

6. Remove the bay leaf. Stir in the cooked brown rice and chopped parsley. Serve the jambalaya immediately.

# Chapter 5 : Dinner

**Lemon Herb Baked Salmon**

Prep Time: 10 minutes
Cook Time: 15 minutes
Total Time: 25 minutes
Serves: 4

**Ingredients:**
- 4 (6 oz) salmon fillets
- 2 tablespoons olive oil
- 2 tablespoons lemon juice
- 2 teaspoons dried oregano
- 2 teaspoons dried basil
- 1 teaspoon garlic powder
- 1/2 teaspoon salt
- 1/4 teaspoon black pepper

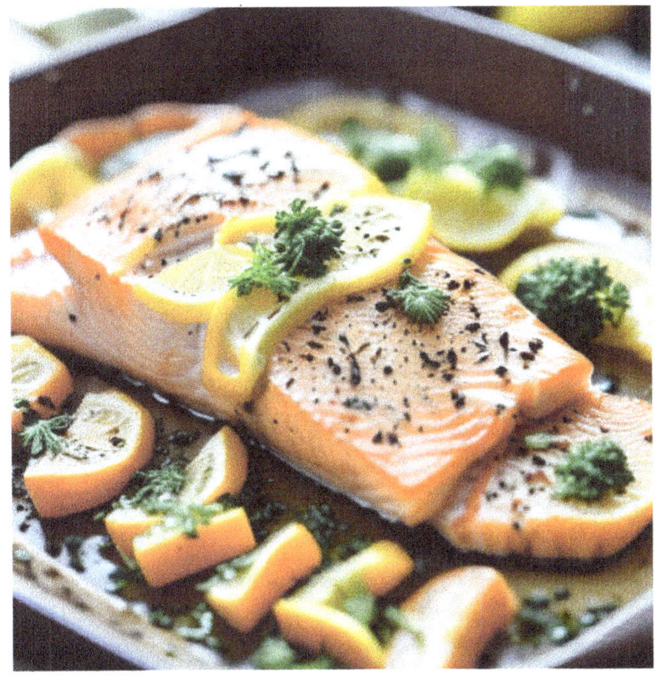

**Directions**:
1. Preheat oven to 400°F. Line a baking sheet with parchment paper or foil.

2. In a small bowl, whisk together the olive oil, lemon juice, oregano, basil, garlic powder, salt, and pepper.

3. Place the salmon fillets on the prepared baking sheet. Brush the tops and sides of the salmon with the lemon herb mixture.

4. Bake for 12-15 minutes, or until the salmon is cooked through and flakes easily with a fork.

5. Serve immediately, garnished with fresh lemon slices if desired.

**Nutrition Facts (per serving):**

Calories: 260
Total Fat: 15g
Saturated Fat: 2.5g
Cholesterol: 80mg
Sodium: 420mg
Total Carbohydrates: 1g
Fiber: 0g
Sugars: 0g
Protein: 27g

**Red Beans and Brown Rice**

Prep Time: 15 minutes
Cook Time: 1 hour
Total Time: 1 hour 15 minutes
Serves: 4

**Ingredients:**
- 1 cup dry red kidney beans, soaked overnight and drained
- 1 tablespoon olive oil
- 1 onion, diced
- 3 cloves garlic, minced
- 1 bell pepper, diced
- 1 celery stalk, diced
- 1 teaspoon dried thyme
- 1 teaspoon dried oregano
- 1/2 teaspoon smoked paprika
- 1/4 teaspoon cayenne pepper (optional)
- 1 bay leaf
- 4 cups low-sodium vegetable or chicken broth
- 1 cup uncooked brown rice
- Salt and black pepper to taste
- Chopped parsley for garnish (optional)

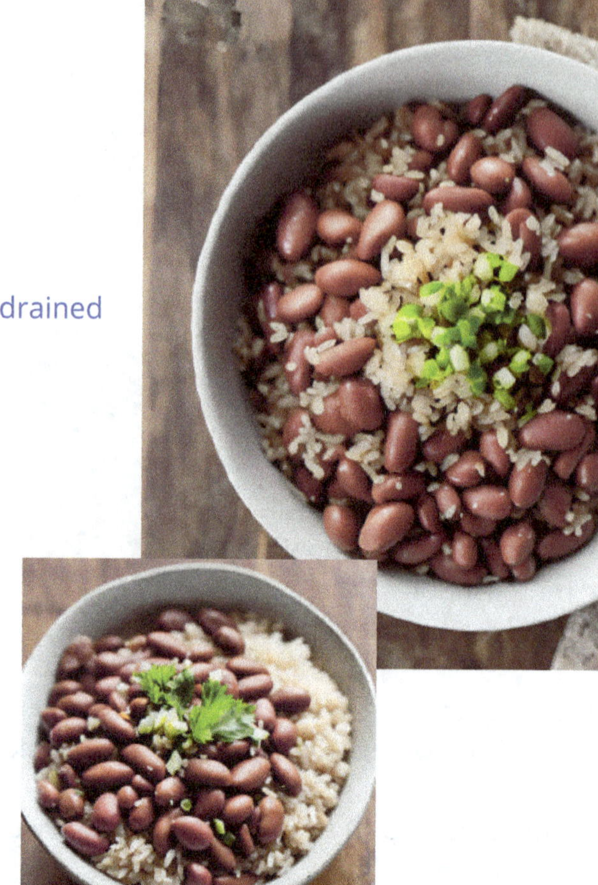

**Directions:**
1. In a large pot, heat the olive oil over medium heat. Add the onion, garlic, bell pepper, and celery. Sauté for 5-7 minutes until softened.
2. Add the soaked and drained red beans, thyme, oregano, smoked paprika, cayenne (if using), and bay leaf. Pour in the broth and stir to combine.
3. Bring the mixture to a boil, then reduce heat to low. Simmer for 45-60 minutes, stirring occasionally, until the beans are very soft.
4. Meanwhile, cook the brown rice according to package instructions.
5. Once the beans are tender, season with salt and pepper to taste.
6. Serve the red beans over the cooked brown rice. Garnish with chopped parsley if desired.

**Nutrition Facts (per serving):**
Calories: 400
Total Fat: 6g
Saturated Fat: 1g
Cholesterol: 0mg
Sodium: 300mg
Total Carbohydrates: 70g
Fiber: 12g
Sugars: 4g
Protein: 16g

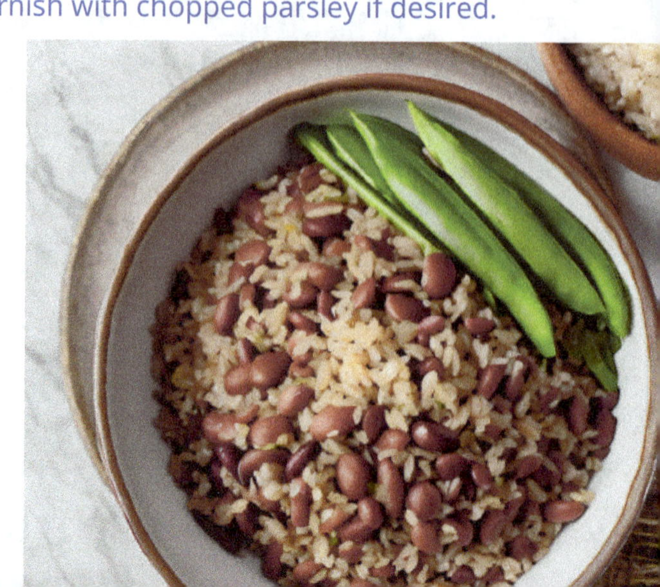

# Chapter 5 : Dinner

**Turkey Meatloaf with Green Beans**

Prep Time: 20 minutes
Cook Time: 1 hour
Total Time: 1 hour 20 minutes
Serves: 6

**Ingredients:**
*Meatloaf:*
- 1 lb ground turkey
- 1 cup breadcrumbs
- 1 egg, beaten
- 1/2 cup milk
- 1/2 onion, finely chopped
- 2 cloves garlic, minced
- 1 tsp dried thyme
- 1 tsp dried oregano
- 1/2 tsp salt
- 1/4 tsp black pepper

*Green Beans:*
- 1 lb fresh green beans, trimmed
- 2 tbsp olive oil
- 2 cloves garlic, minced
- Salt and pepper to taste

*Glaze*:
- 1/2 cup ketchup
- 2 tbsp brown sugar
- 1 tbsp Dijon mustard

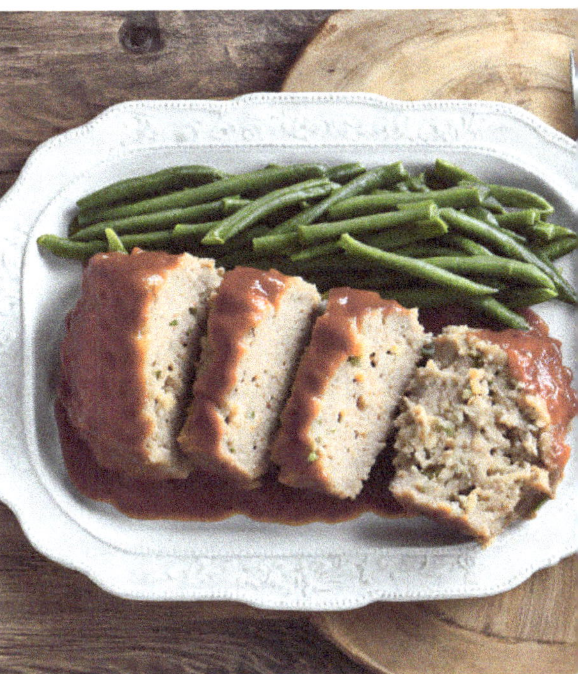
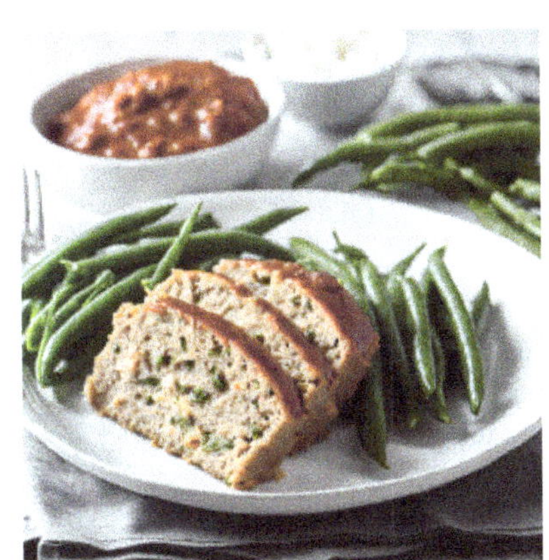
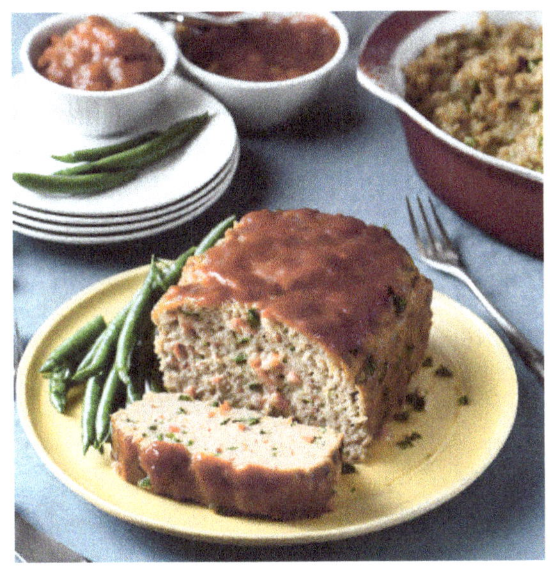

**Directions**:
1. Preheat oven to 375°F. Grease a 9x5 inch loaf pan.
2. In a large bowl, combine all the meatloaf ingredients and mix well. Transfer to the prepared loaf pan and shape into a loaf.
3. In a small bowl, mix together the glaze ingredients. Spread half the glaze over the top of the meatloaf.
4. Bake for 45 minutes. Remove from oven and spread the remaining glaze over the top. Bake for an additional 15 minutes.
5. While the meatloaf is baking, prepare the green beans. In a large skillet, heat the olive oil over medium heat. Add the garlic and sauté for 1 minute.
6. Add the green beans and season with salt and pepper. Cook for 10-12 minutes, stirring occasionally, until beans are tender.
7. Let the meatloaf rest for 5 minutes before slicing. Serve the meatloaf with the green beans on the side.

# Chapter 6 : Snacks

**Spicy Baked Okra Chips**

Prep Time: 10 minutes
Cook Time: 20 minutes
Total Time: 30 minutes
Serves: 4

**Ingredients:**
- 1 lb fresh okra, washed and
sliced into 1/2-inch thick rounds
- 2 tablespoons olive oil
- 1 teaspoon smoked paprika
- 1 teaspoon garlic powder
- 1/2 teaspoon cayenne pepper (or to taste)
- 1/2 teaspoon salt

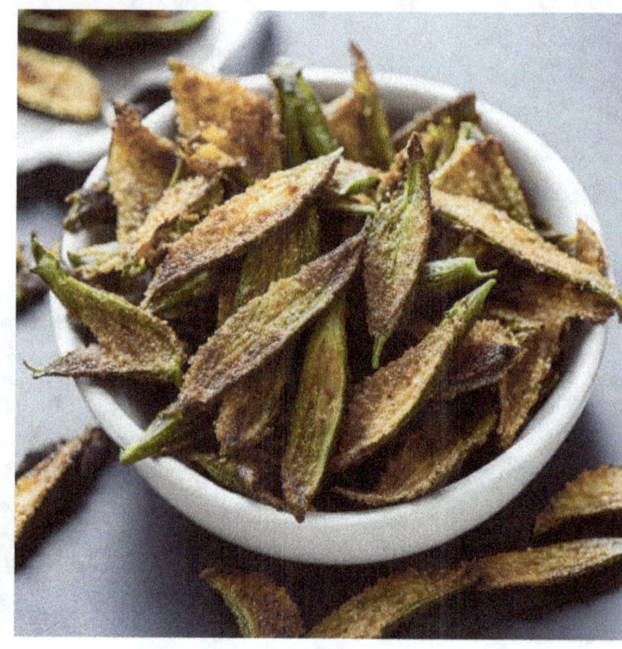

**Directions**:

1. Preheat oven to 400°F. Line a large baking sheet with parchment paper.

2. In a large bowl, toss the sliced okra with the olive oil, smoked paprika, garlic powder, cayenne pepper, and salt until evenly coated.

3. Spread the okra in a single layer on the prepared baking sheet.

4. Bake for 15-20 minutes, flipping the okra halfway through, until crispy and lightly browned.

5. Remove from oven and let cool for 5 minutes before serving.

**Nutrition Facts (per serving):**
Calories: 80
Total Fat: 5g
Saturated Fat: 1g
Cholesterol: 0mg
Sodium: 240mg
Total Carbohydrates: 8g
Fiber: 3g
Sugars: 2g
Protein: 2g

# Chapter 6 : Snacks

**Sweet Potato Fries**

Prep Time: 10 minutes
Cook Time: 25 minutes
Total Time: 35 minutes
Serves: 4

**Ingredients**:
- 2 lbs sweet potatoes, peeled
and cut into 1/2-inch thick fry shapes
- 2 tablespoons olive oil
- 1 teaspoon garlic powder
- 1 teaspoon paprika
- 1/2 teaspoon salt
- 1/4 teaspoon black pepper

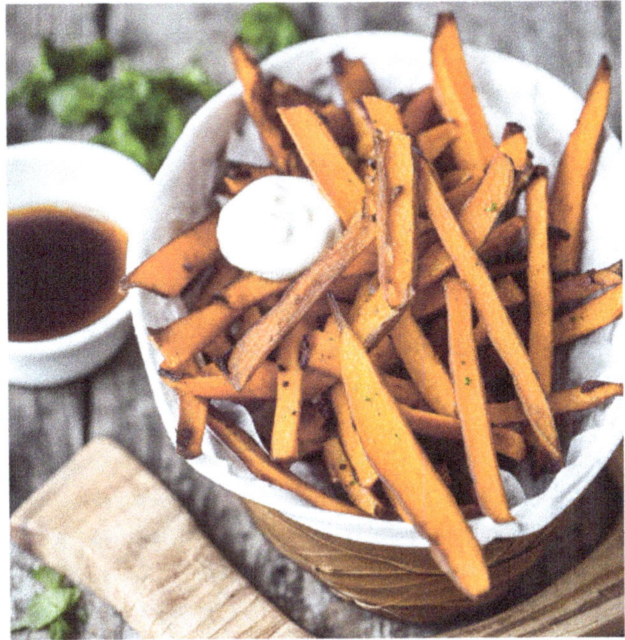

**Directions:**
1. Preheat oven to 400°F. Line a large baking sheet with parchment paper.

2. In a large bowl, toss the sweet potato fries with the olive oil, garlic powder, paprika, salt, and pepper until evenly coated.

3. Spread the fries in a single layer on the prepared baking sheet, making sure they are not touching each other.

4. Bake for 20-25 minutes, flipping the fries halfway through, until golden brown and crispy.

5. Remove from oven and serve hot.

**Nutrition Facts (per serving):**
Calories: 160
Total Fat: 6g
Saturated Fat: 1g
Cholesterol: 0mg
Sodium: 260mg
Total Carbohydrates: 25g
Fiber: 4g
Sugars: 6g
Protein: 2g

# Chapter 6 : Snacks

**Hummus with Veggie Sticks**

Prep Time: 15 minutes
Total Time: 15 minutes
Serves: 4

**Ingredients:**
*Hummus:*
- 1 (15 oz) can chickpeas, drained and rinsed
- 2 tablespoons tahini
- 2 tablespoons lemon juice
- 1 garlic clove, minced
- 2 tablespoons olive oil
- 1/4 teaspoon ground cumin
- 1/4 teaspoon paprika
- Salt and pepper to taste

*Veggie Sticks:*
- 1 cucumber, cut into sticks
- 1 red bell pepper, cut into sticks
- 1 cup baby carrots
- 1 cup cherry tomatoes

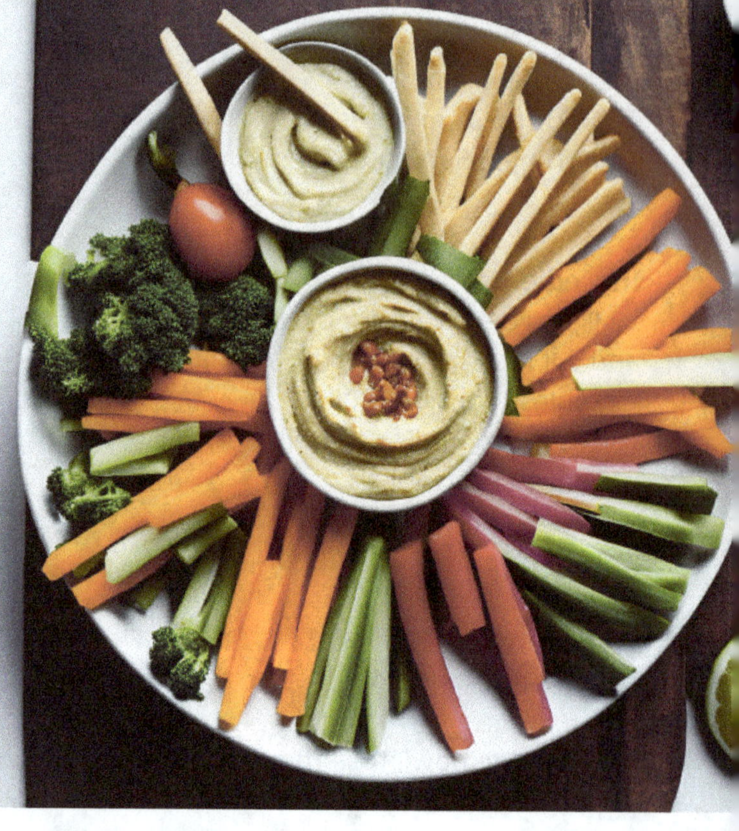

**Directions:**

1. In a food processor, combine all the hummus ingredients and blend until smooth and creamy. Taste and adjust seasoning as needed.

2. Transfer the hummus to a serving bowl.

3. Arrange the veggie sticks around the hummus in a platter or on a plate.

4. Serve the hummus with the fresh veggie sticks for dipping.

Nutrition Facts (per serving):
Calories: 180
Total Fat: 11g
Saturated Fat: 1.5g
Cholesterol: 0mg
Sodium: 300mg
Total Carbohydrates: 17g
Fiber: 5g
Sugars: 4g
Protein: 6g

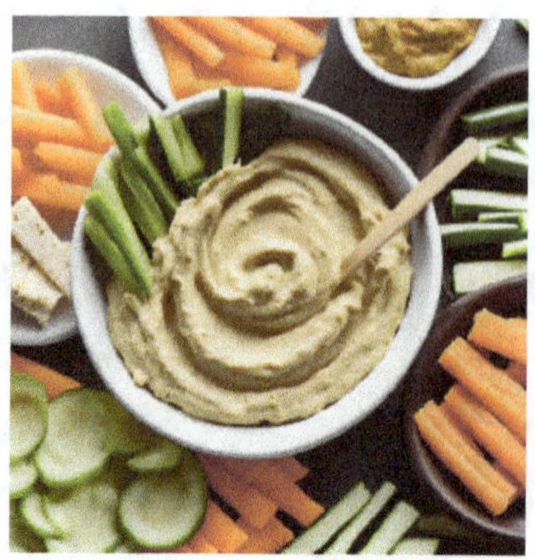

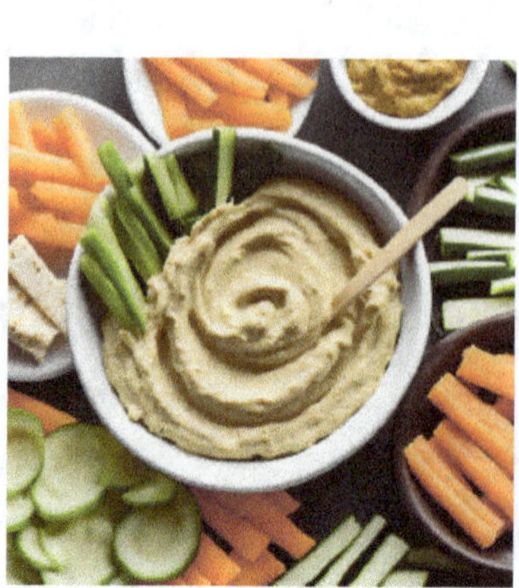

# Chapter 6 : Snacks

## Baked Plantain Chips

Prep Time: 10 minutes
Cook Time: 20 minutes
Total Time: 30 minutes
Serves: 4

### Ingredients:
- 2 green plantains, peeled and sliced into 1/4-inch thick rounds
- 2 tablespoons olive oil
- 1 teaspoon salt
- 1/2 teaspoon ground cumin (optional)
- 1/4 teaspoon chili powder (optional)

### Directions:

1. Preheat oven to 400°F. Line two baking sheets with parchment paper.

2. In a large bowl, toss the plantain slices with the olive oil, salt, and any optional spices until evenly coated.

3. Arrange the plantain slices in a single layer on the prepared baking sheets, making sure they are not overlapping.

4. Bake for 10 minutes, then flip the slices and bake for another 10-12 minutes, until golden brown and crispy.

5. Remove from oven and let cool for 5 minutes before serving.

### Nutrition Facts (per serving):
Calories: 150
Total Fat: 6g
Saturated Fat: 1g
Cholesterol: 0mg
Sodium: 360mg
Total Carbohydrates: 23g
Fiber: 2g
Sugars: 3g
Protein: 1g

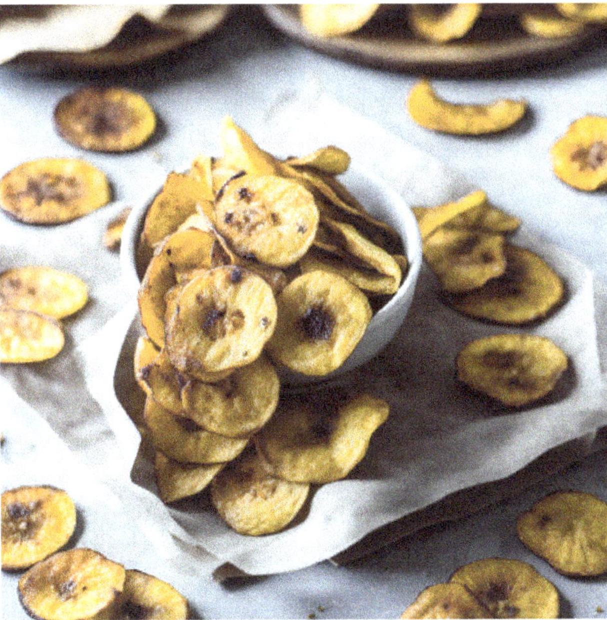

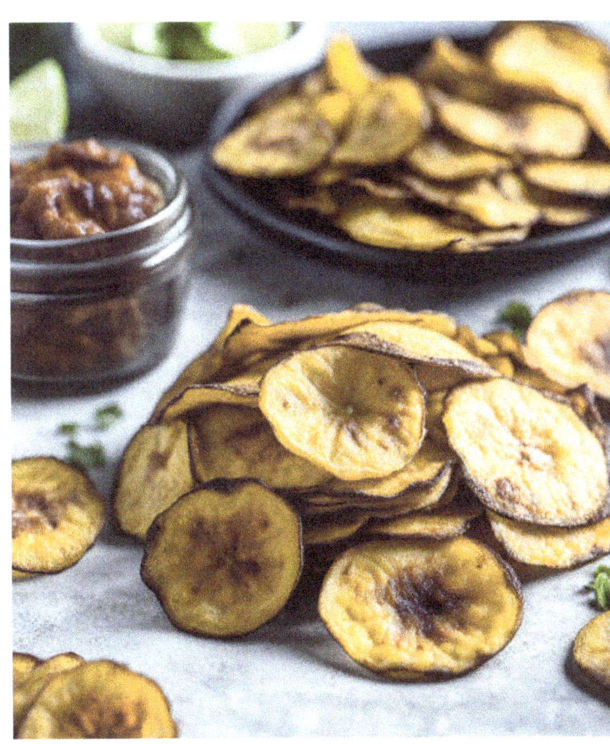

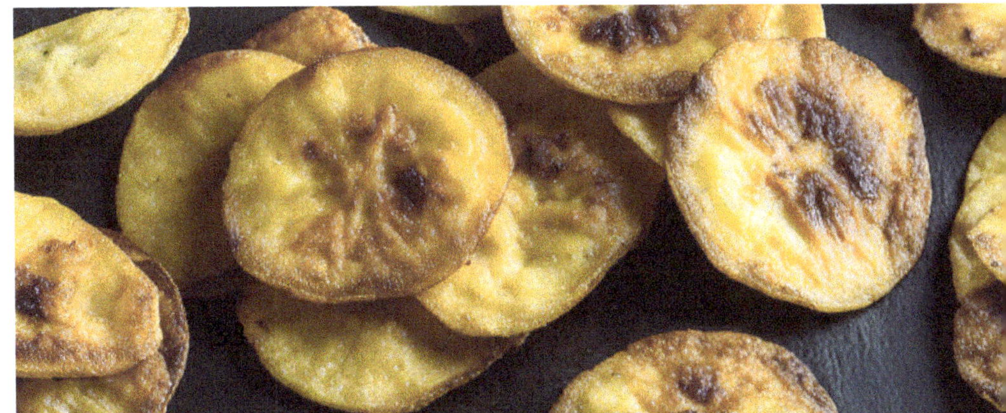

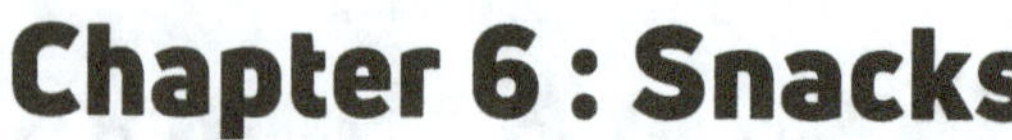

# Chapter 6 : Snacks

### Low-Sugar Pecan Bars

Prep Time: 15 minutes
Cook Time: 25 minutes
Total Time: 40 minutes
Serves: 16 bars

**Ingredients**:
Crust:
- 1 cup almond flour
- 1/4 cup coconut flour
- 1/4 cup unsweetened shredded coconut
- 1/4 cup melted coconut oil
- 1 tablespoon honey

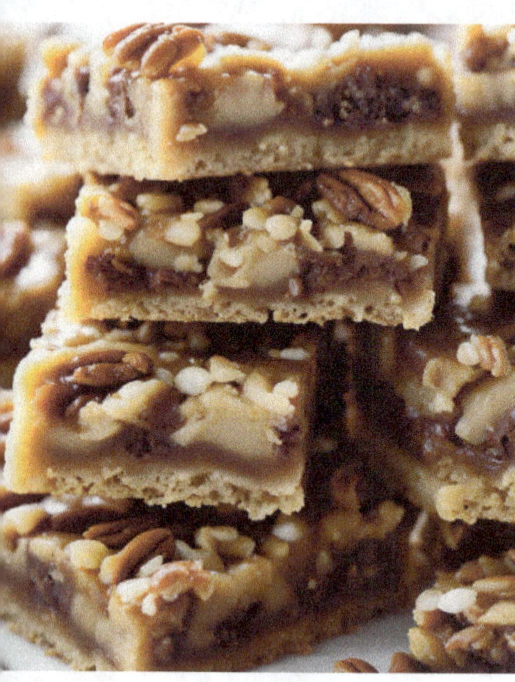

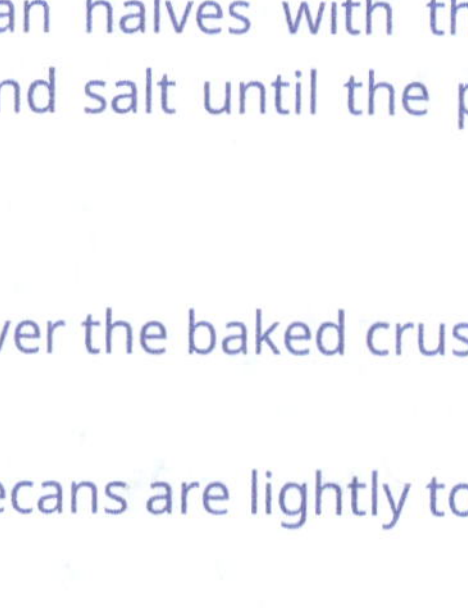

Filling:
- 2 cups pecan halves
- 1/4 cup honey
- 1 tablespoon coconut oil, melted
- 1 teaspoon vanilla extract
- 1/4 teaspoon salt

**Directions**:
1. Preheat oven to 350°F. Line an 8x8 inch baking pan with parchment paper.

2. In a medium bowl, mix together the almond flour, coconut flour, shredded coconut, melted coconut oil, and 1 tablespoon honey until well combined. Press the mixture evenly into the bottom of the prepared pan.

3. Bake the crust for 10 minutes, then remove from oven and let cool slightly.

4. In a medium bowl, toss the pecan halves with the 1/4 cup honey, melted coconut oil, vanilla, and salt until the pecans are evenly coated.

5. Spread the pecan mixture evenly over the baked crust.

6. Bake for 15-20 minutes, until the pecans are lightly toasted.

7. Allow the bars to cool completely in the pan before lifting out using the parchment paper. Cut into 16 bars.

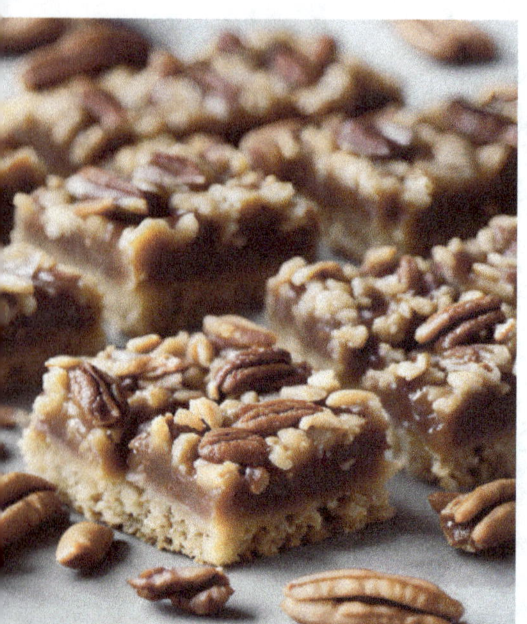

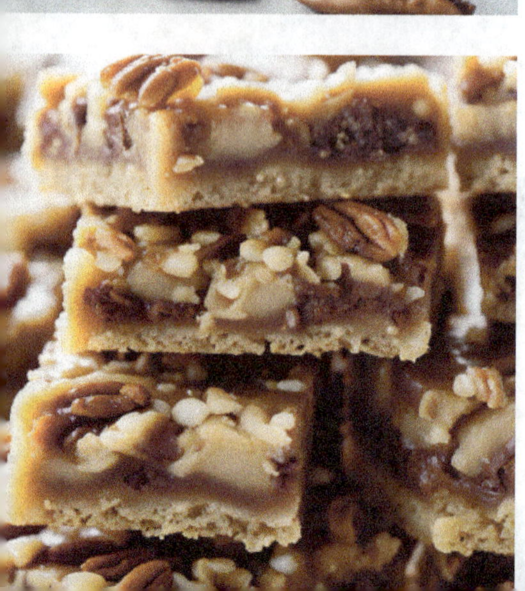

# Chapter 6 : Snacks

## Cucumber and Tomato Salad

Prep Time: 15 minutes
Total Time: 15 minutes
Serves: 4

**Ingredients:**
- 2 cucumbers, sliced
- 2 cups cherry tomatoes, halved
- 1/2 red onion, thinly sliced
- 1/4 cup fresh basil leaves, chopped
- 2 tablespoons olive oil
- 2 tablespoons red wine vinegar
- 1 teaspoon Dijon mustard
- 1 garlic clove, minced
- 1/4 teaspoon salt
- 1/4 teaspoon black pepper

**Instructions:**

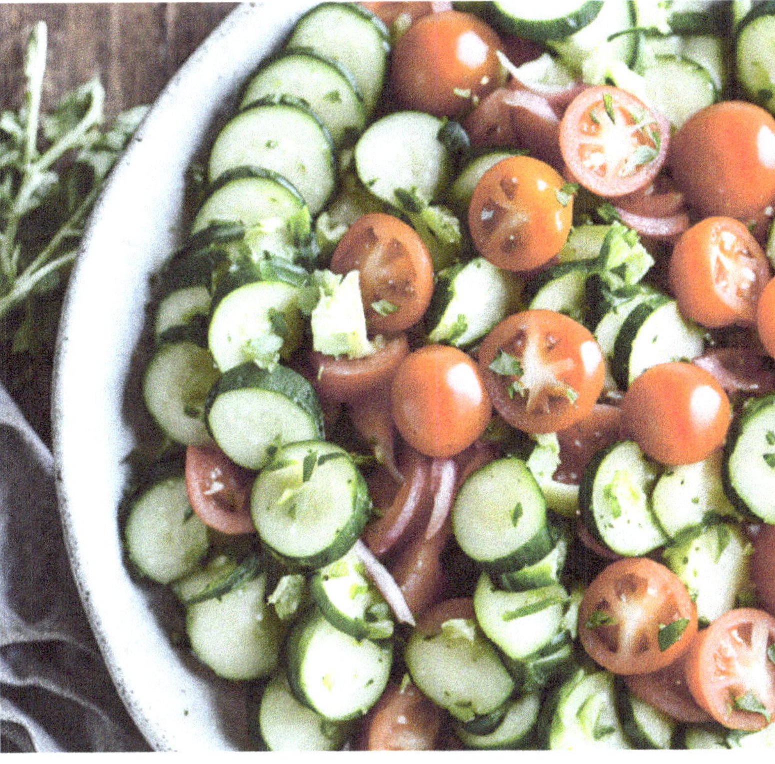

1. In a large bowl, combine the sliced cucumbers, halved cherry tomatoes, sliced red onion, and chopped basil.

2. In a small bowl, whisk together the olive oil, red wine vinegar, Dijon mustard, minced garlic, salt, and black pepper.

3. Pour the dressing over the cucumber and tomato mixture and toss gently to coat.

4. Refrigerate for at least 30 minutes to allow the flavors to meld. Serve chilled or at room temperature.

Nutrition Facts (per serving):
Calories: 90
Total Fat: 6g
Saturated Fat: 1g
Cholesterol: 0mg
Sodium: 200mg
Total Carbohydrates: 9g
Fiber: 2g
Sugars: 5g
Protein: 2g

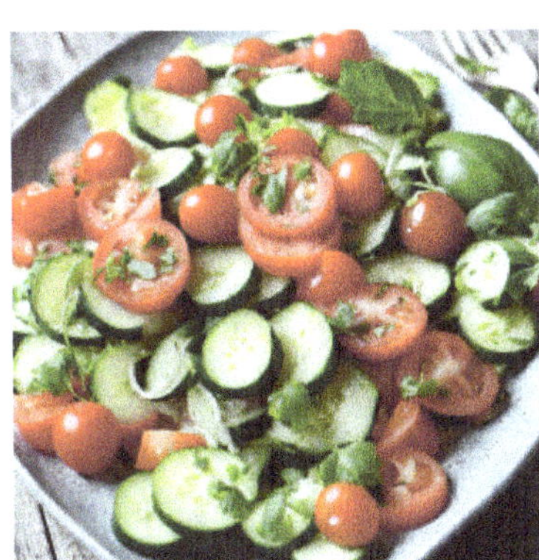

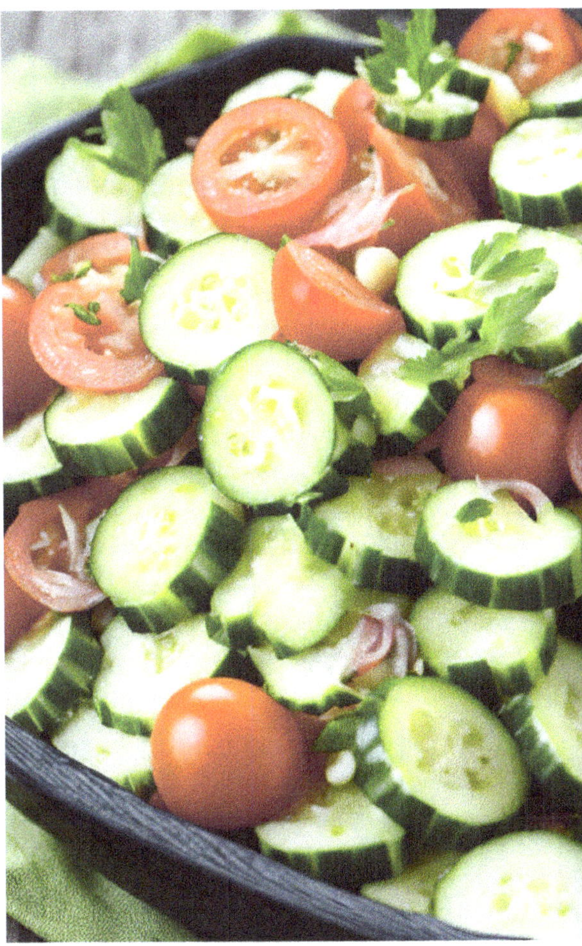

# Chapter 6 : Snacks

**Greek Yogurt with Fresh Berries**

Prep Time: 5 minutes
Total Time: 5 minutes
Serves: 2

**Ingredients:**
- 1 cup plain Greek yogurt
- 1 cup mixed fresh berries (such as strawberries, blueberries, raspberries)
- 1 tablespoon honey (optional)
- 1 teaspoon lemon zest (optional)

**Instructions:**

1. Divide the Greek yogurt between two serving bowls or glasses.

2. Top each serving with about 1/2 cup of the mixed fresh berries.

3. Drizzle 1/2 tablespoon of honey over each serving, if desired.

4. Sprinkle 1/2 teaspoon of lemon zest over each serving, if desired. Serve immediately.

**Nutrition Facts (per serving):**
Calories: 150
Total Fat: 4g
Saturated Fat: 2g
Cholesterol: 15mg
Sodium: 55mg
Total Carbohydrates: 18g
Fiber: 3g
Sugars: 14g
Protein: 15g

This simple and healthy Greek yogurt parfait is a great way to start the day or enjoy as a light snack. The combination of creamy Greek yogurt, fresh berries, and a touch of honey or lemon zest provides a delicious and nutritious treat.

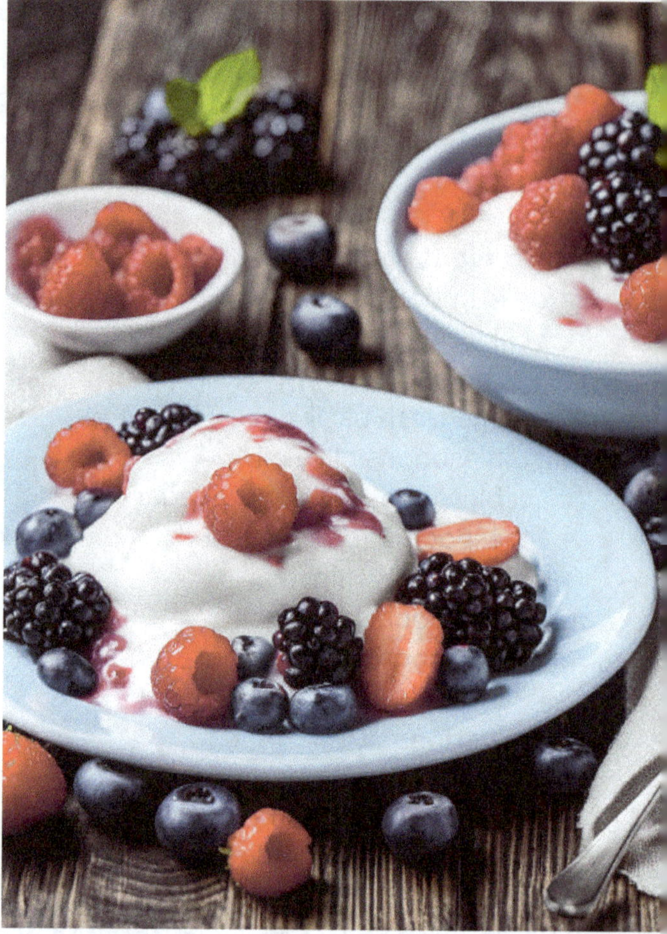

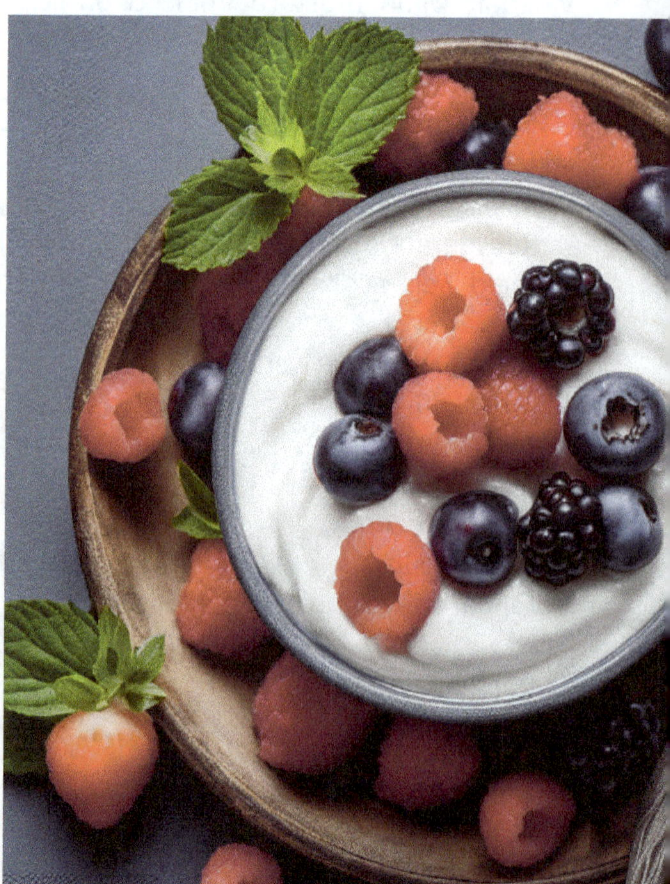

# Chapter 7 : Desserts

**Sugar-Free Sweet Potato Pie**

Prep Time: 20 minutes
Cook Time: 1 hour
Total Time: 1 hour 20 minutes
Serves: 8

**Ingredients:**
Crust:
- 1 1/4 cups almond flour
- 2 tablespoons coconut oil, melted
- 1 tablespoon water

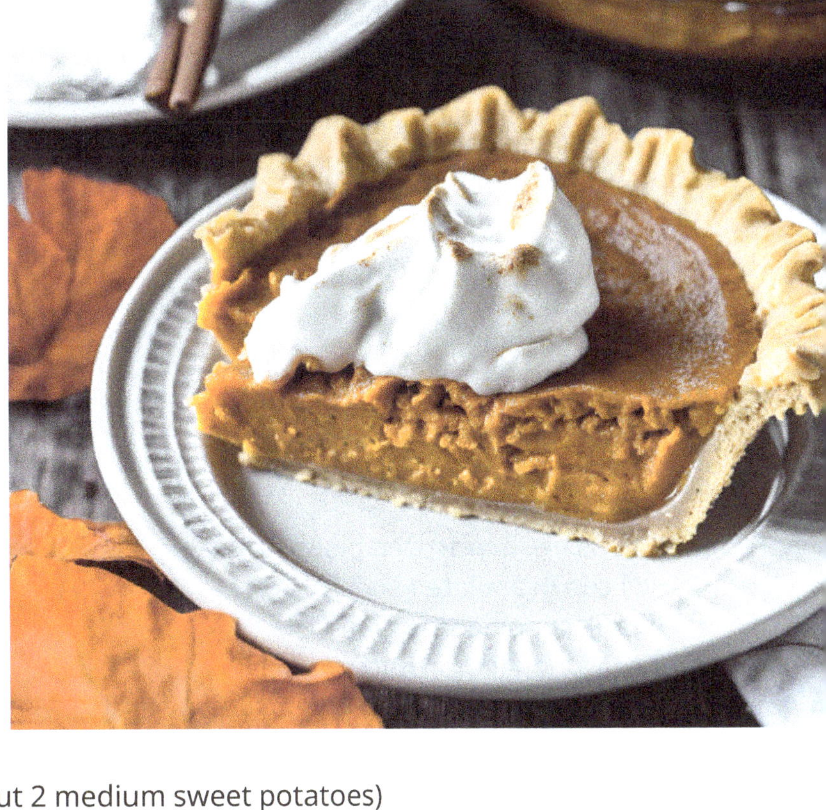

Filling:
- 2 cups mashed cooked sweet potatoes (about 2 medium sweet potatoes)
- 3 large eggs
- 1/2 cup unsweetened almond milk
- 1/4 cup granulated erythritol or other zero-calorie sweetener
- 1 teaspoon ground cinnamon
- 1/2 teaspoon ground ginger
- 1/4 teaspoon ground nutmeg
- 1/4 teaspoon salt

**Instructions**:
1. Preheat oven to 350°F. Grease a 9-inch pie plate.
2. Make the crust: In a medium bowl, mix together the almond flour, melted coconut oil, and water until a dough forms. Press the dough evenly into the bottom and up the sides of the prepared pie plate.
3. Make the filling: In a large bowl, whisk together the mashed sweet potatoes, eggs, almond milk, erythritol, cinnamon, ginger, nutmeg, and salt until well combined.
4. Pour the filling into the prepared crust.
5. Bake for 50-60 minutes, until the center is set. Allow the pie to cool completely before slicing.
6. Serve chilled or at room temperature.

**Nutrition Facts (per slice):**
Calories: 190
Total Fat: 13g
Saturated Fat: 5g
Cholesterol: 95mg
Sodium: 160mg
Total Carbohydrates: 14g
Fiber: 3g
Sugars: 2g
Protein: 6g

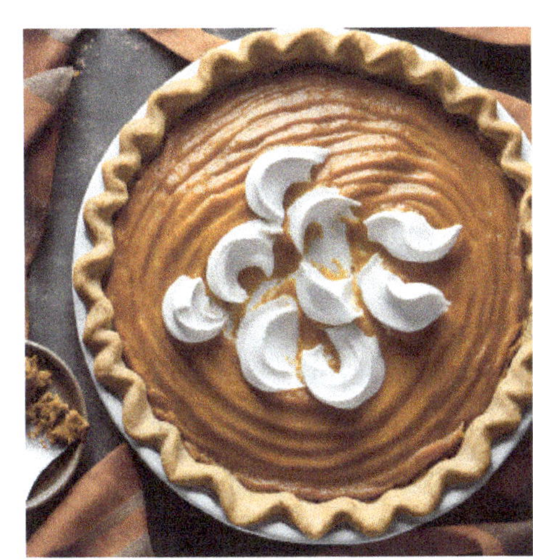

# Chapter 7 : Desserts

**Blueberry Cobbler**

Prep Time: 15 minutes
Cook Time: 35 minutes
Total Time: 50 minutes
Serves: 6

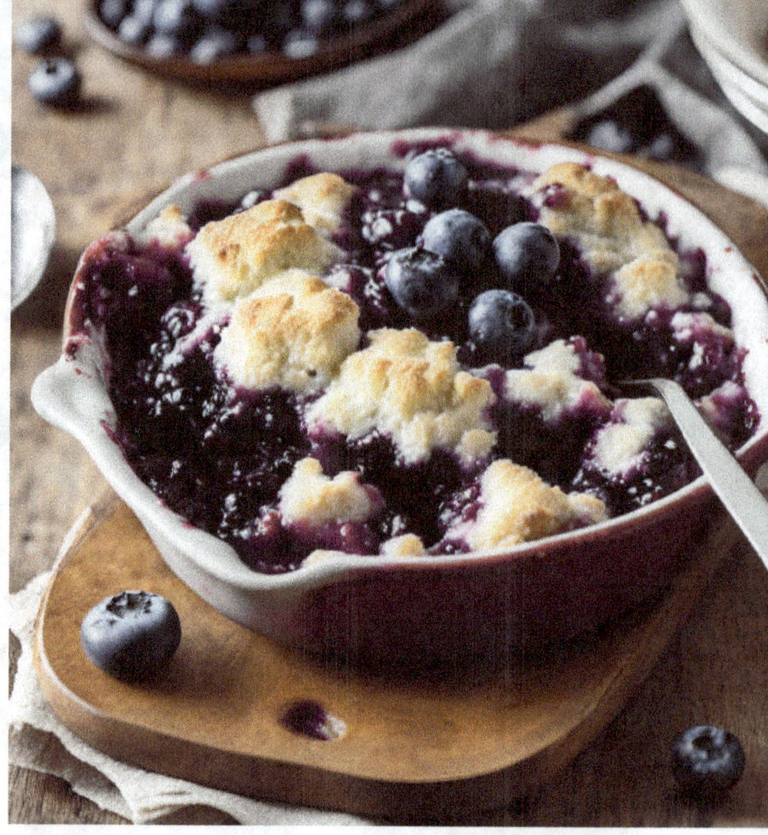

**Ingredients:**
Filling:
- 4 cups fresh or frozen blueberries
- 1/4 cup granulated sugar
- 1 tablespoon cornstarch
- 1 teaspoon lemon juice
- 1/4 teaspoon ground cinnamon

Topping:
- 1 cup all-purpose flour
- 1/4 cup granulated sugar
- 2 teaspoons baking powder
- 1/4 teaspoon salt
- 5 tablespoons cold unsalted butter, cubed
- 1/2 cup milk

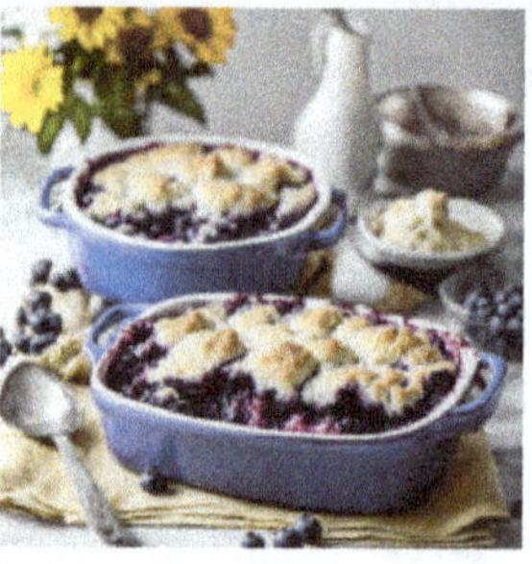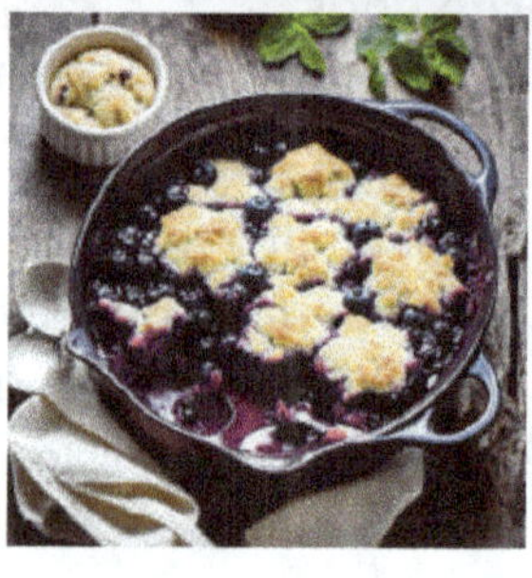

**Instructions**:
1. Preheat oven to 375°F. Grease an 8x8 inch baking dish.
2. Make the filling: In a large bowl, gently toss together the blueberries, 1/4 cup sugar, cornstarch, lemon juice, and cinnamon. Pour the filling into the prepared baking dish.
3. Make the topping: In a medium bowl, whisk together the flour, 1/4 cup sugar, baking powder, and salt. Cut in the cold butter using a pastry blender or two forks until the mixture resembles coarse crumbs. Stir in the milk just until combined.
4. Drop the topping batter by large spoonfuls onto the blueberry filling, leaving some space between the spoonfuls.
5. Bake for 30-35 minutes, until the topping is golden brown and the filling is bubbling.
6. Allow to cool for 15 minutes before serving. Serve warm, with a scoop of vanilla ice cream if desired.

Nutrition Facts (per serving):
Calories: 280
Total Fat: 9g
Saturated Fat: 5g
Cholesterol: 20mg
Sodium: 260mg
Total Carbohydrates: 47g
Fiber: 3g
Sugars: 24g

# Chapter 7 : Desserts

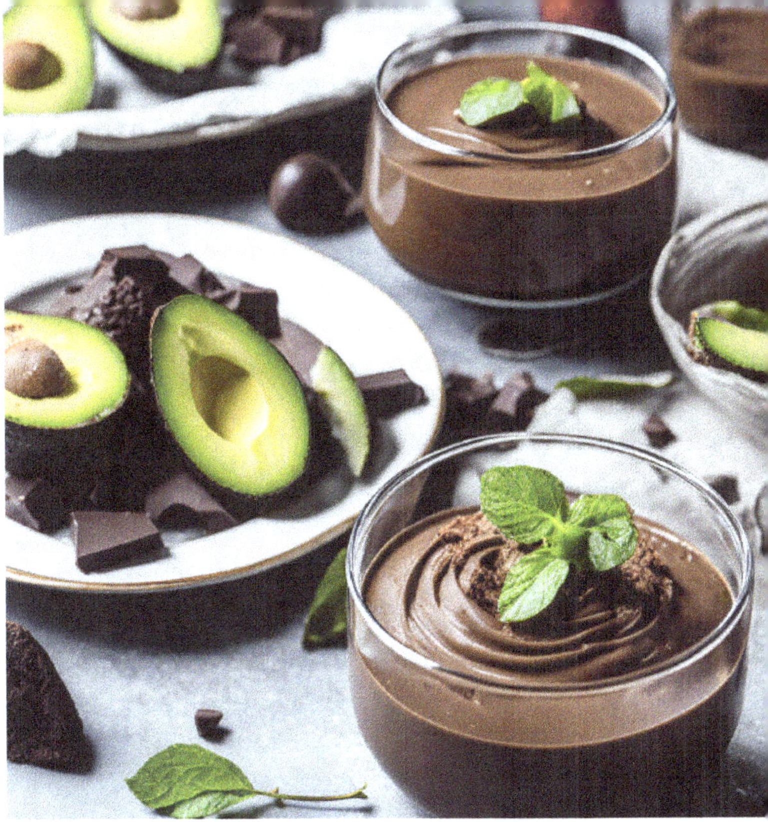

**Chocolate Avocado Mousse**

Prep Time: 10 minutes
Chill Time: 2 hours
Total Time: 2 hours 10 minutes
Serves: 4

**Ingredients**:
- 2 ripe avocados, pitted and flesh scooped out
- 1/2 cup unsweetened cocoa powder
- 1/4 cup maple syrup
- 1 teaspoon vanilla extract
- 1/4 teaspoon sea salt

**Instructions**:

1. In a food processor or high-powered blender, combine the avocado flesh, cocoa powder, maple syrup, vanilla, and salt. Blend until completely smooth and creamy, scraping down the sides as needed.

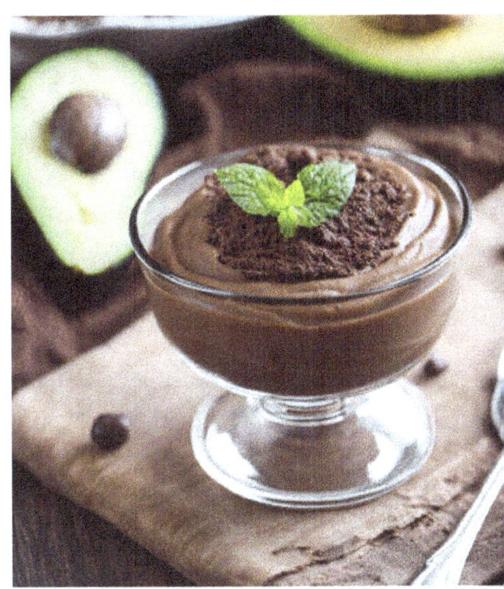

2. Transfer the chocolate avocado mousse to a bowl or individual serving dishes. Cover and refrigerate for at least 2 hours, or until chilled and set.

3. Serve chilled, garnished with fresh berries, shaved dark chocolate, or a dollop of whipped cream if desired.

**Nutrition Facts (per serving):**
Calories: 200
Total Fat: 14g
Saturated Fat: 2g
Cholesterol: 0mg
Sodium: 100mg
Total Carbohydrates: 20g
Fiber: 7g
Sugars: 10g
Protein: 4g

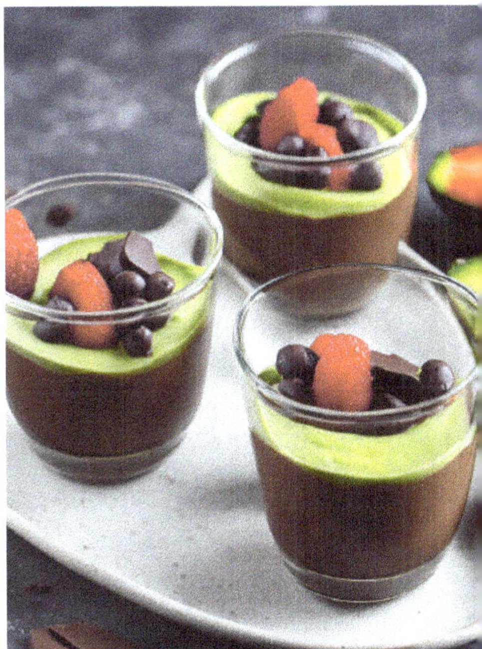

This rich and creamy chocolate avocado mousse is a healthy and delicious dessert. The avocado provides a smooth, creamy texture while the cocoa powder and maple syrup give it a deep chocolate flavor. It's a great option for those looking for a low-sugar, nutrient-dense treat.

# Chapter 7 : Desserts

**Peach Crisp**

Prep Time: 15 minutes
Cook Time: 35 minutes
Total Time: 50 minutes
Serves: 6

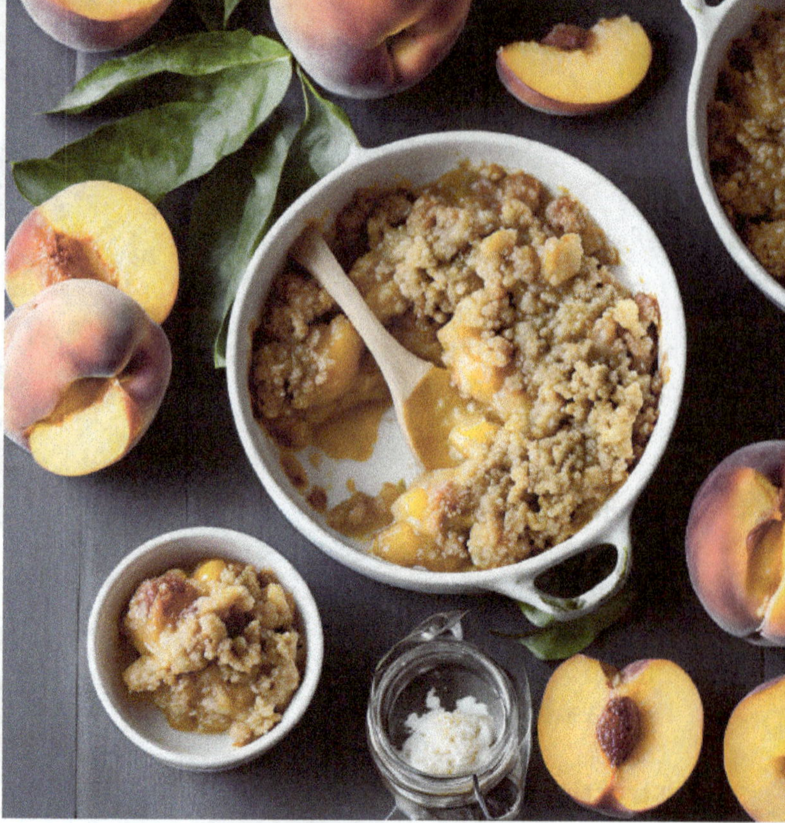

## Ingredients:

Filling:
- 6 cups sliced fresh or frozen peaches
- 2 tablespoons granulated sugar
- 1 tablespoon cornstarch
- 1 teaspoon lemon juice

Topping:
- 1 cup old-fashioned oats
- 1/2 cup all-purpose flour
- 1/2 cup packed brown sugar
- 1/2 cup chopped pecans
- 1/2 teaspoon ground cinnamon
- 1/4 teaspoon salt
- 6 tablespoons cold unsalted butter, cubed

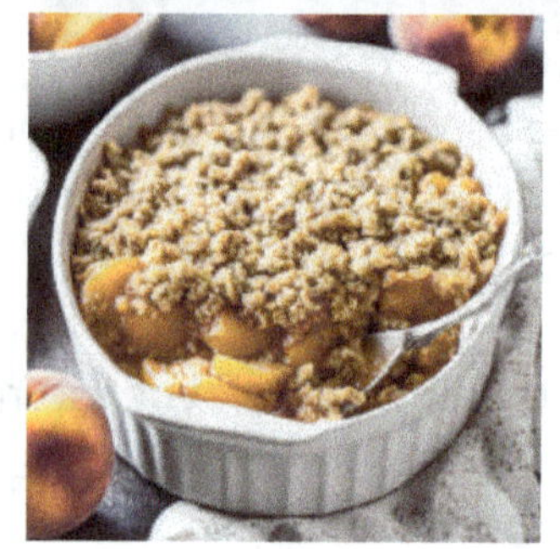
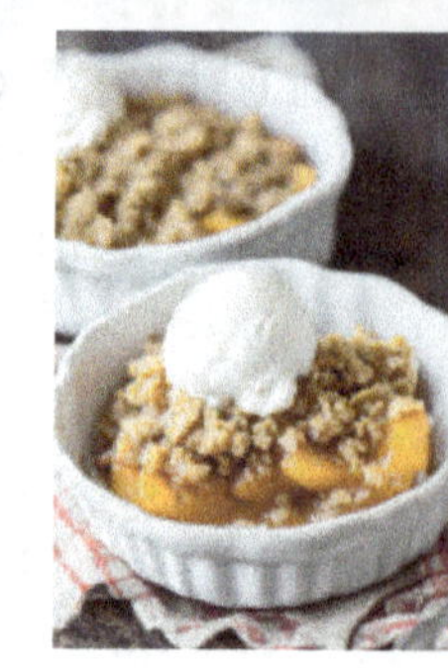

## Instructions:

1. Preheat oven to 375°F. Grease an 8x8 inch baking dish.
2. Make the filling: In a large bowl, gently toss together the peach slices, granulated sugar, cornstarch, and lemon juice. Pour the filling into the prepared baking dish.
3. Make the topping: In a medium bowl, combine the oats, flour, brown sugar, pecans, cinnamon, and salt. Cut in the cold butter using a pastry blender or two forks until the mixture resembles coarse crumbs.
4. Sprinkle the oat topping evenly over the peach filling.
5. Bake for 30-35 minutes, until the topping is golden brown and the filling is bubbling.
6. Allow to cool for 15 minutes before serving. Serve warm, with a scoop of vanilla ice cream if desired.

Nutrition Facts (per serving):
Calories: 340
Total Fat: 15g
Saturated Fat: 6g
Cholesterol: 20mg
Sodium: 120mg
Total Carbohydrates: 50g
Fiber: 4g
Sugars: 32g
Protein: 4g

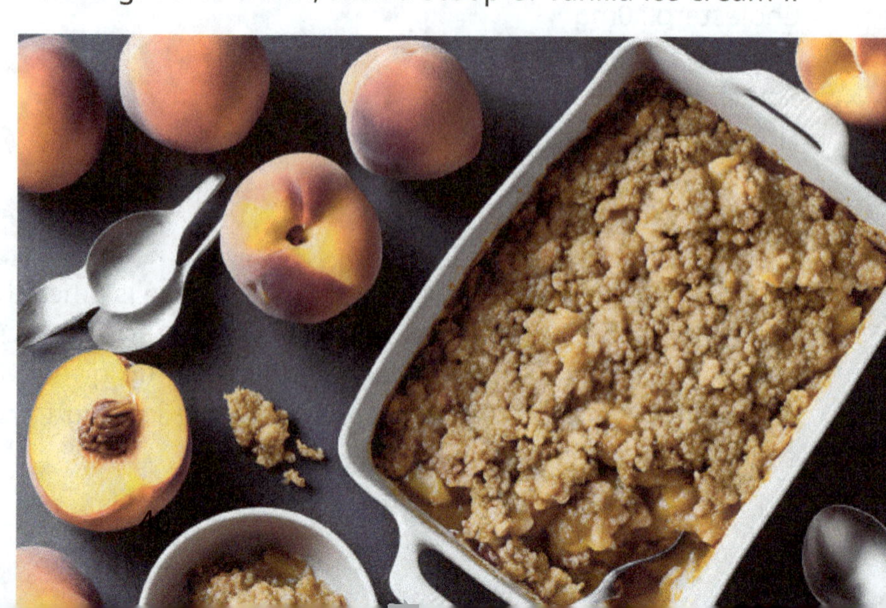

# Chapter 7 : Desserts

**Vanilla Bean Pudding**

Prep Time: 15 minutes
Cook Time: 15 minutes
Chill Time: 2 hours
Total Time: 2 hours 30 minutes
Serves: 4

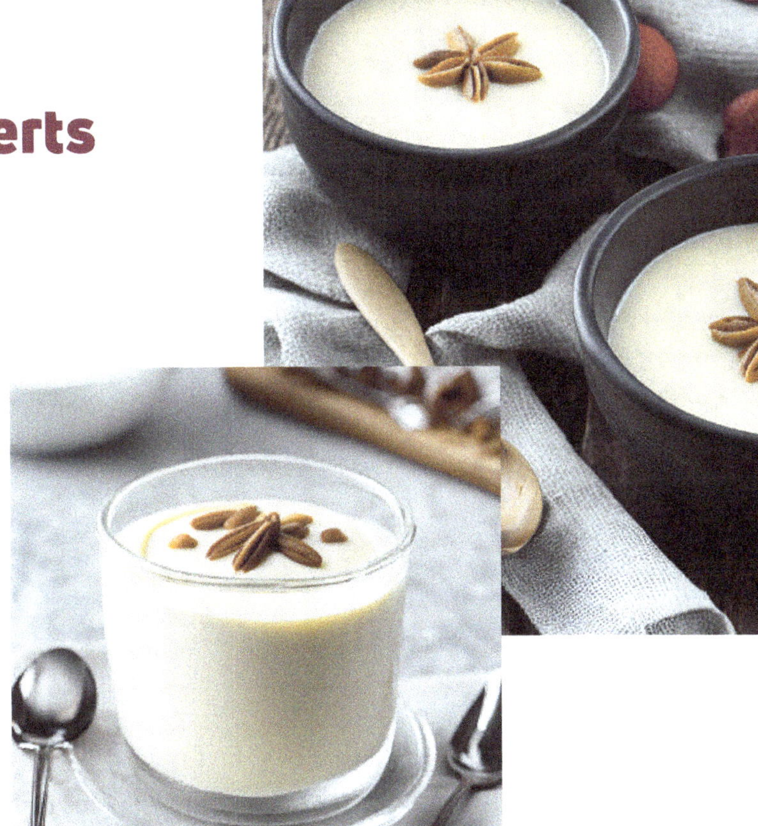

**Ingredients:**
- 2 cups whole milk
- 1 vanilla bean, split lengthwise
- 1/4 cup granulated sugar
- 2 tablespoons cornstarch
- 2 large egg yolks
- 1 teaspoon vanilla extract
- Pinch of salt

**Instructions:**
1. In a medium saucepan, combine the milk and vanilla bean. Heat over medium, stirring occasionally, until steaming and bubbles start to form around the edges, about 5 minutes.
2. In a medium bowl, whisk together the sugar, cornstarch, and egg yolks until smooth.
3. Slowly pour 1/2 cup of the hot milk mixture into the egg yolk mixture, whisking constantly. Then pour the egg mixture back into the saucepan with the remaining milk.
4. Cook over medium heat, stirring constantly with a wooden spoon or heatproof spatula, until the mixture thickens and bubbles, about 5-7 minutes.
5. Remove from heat and stir in the vanilla extract and a pinch of salt.
6. Strain the pudding through a fine-mesh sieve into a clean bowl. Cover the surface with plastic wrap to prevent a skin from forming. Refrigerate for at least 2 hours, until chilled and set.
7. Serve chilled, garnished with fresh berries or a dollop of whipped cream if desired.

Nutrition Facts (per serving):
Calories: 190
Total Fat: 8g
Saturated Fat: 4g
Cholesterol: 110mg
Sodium: 75mg
Total Carbohydrates: 24g
Fiber: 0g
Sugars: 19g
Protein: 6g

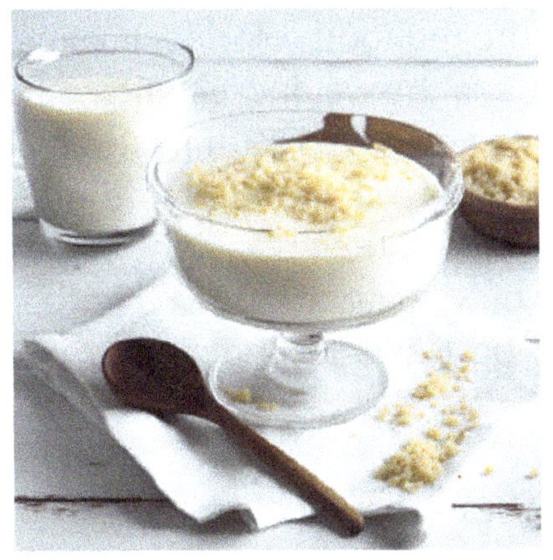
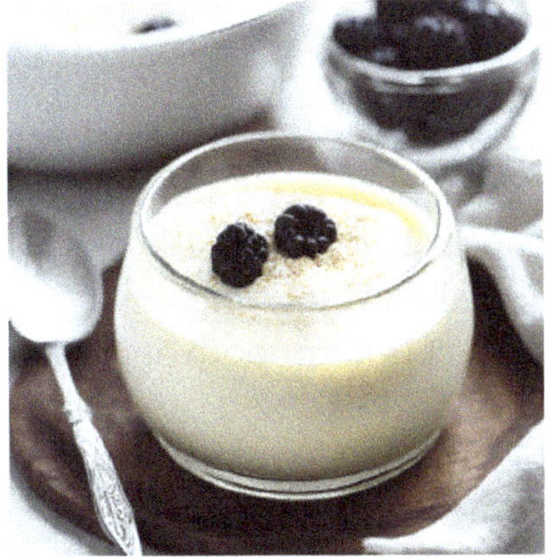

This rich and creamy vanilla bean pudding is a classic, comforting dessert. The use of a vanilla bean gives it an intense vanilla flavor, while the egg yolks provide a luxurious texture. It's a perfect make-ahead treat for any occasion.

# Chapter 7 : Desserts

**Low-Sugar Red Velvet Cupcakes**

Prep Time: 20 minutes
Cook Time: 18 minutes
Total Time: 38 minutes
Serves: 12 cupcakes

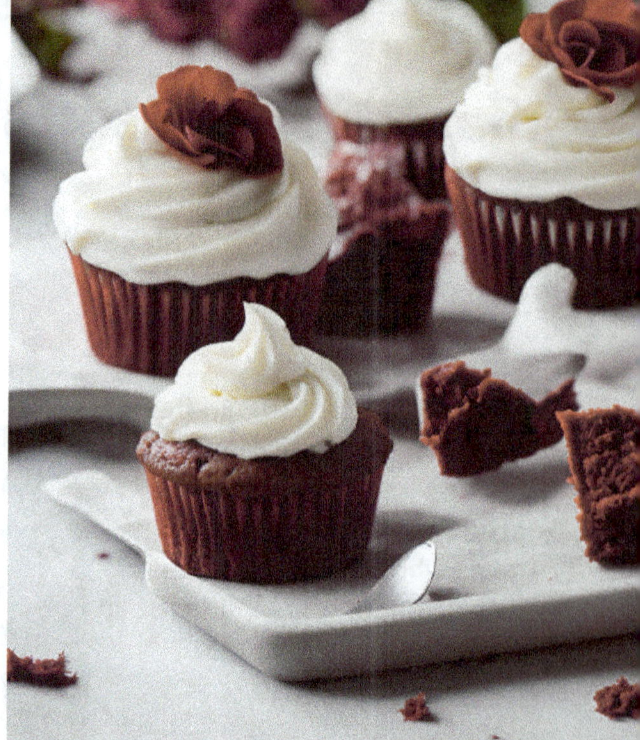

**Ingredients:**
Cupcakes:
- 1 cup all-purpose flour
- 2 tablespoons unsweetened cocoa powder
- 1 teaspoon baking soda
- 1/4 teaspoon salt
- 1/2 cup unsweetened applesauce
- 1/4 cup granulated erythritol or other zero-calorie sweetener
- 1 large egg
- 1 teaspoon vanilla extract
- 1 tablespoon red food coloring (optional)

Cream Cheese Frosting:
- 4 ounces reduced-fat cream cheese, softened
- 1/4 cup powdered erythritol or other zero-calorie sweetener
- 1 teaspoon vanilla extract
- 1-2 tablespoons unsweetened almond milk (if needed)

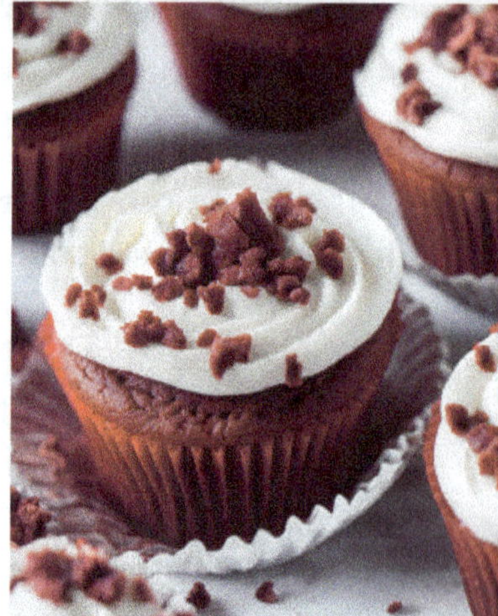

**Instructions**:
1. Preheat oven to 350°F. Line a 12-cup muffin tin with paper liners.
2. In a medium bowl, whisk together the flour, cocoa powder, baking soda, and salt.
3. In a separate bowl, beat the applesauce and granulated erythritol until well combined. Beat in the egg and vanilla extract. Stir in the red food coloring, if using.
4. Gradually add the dry ingredients to the wet ingredients, mixing just until combined.
5. Divide the batter evenly among the prepared muffin cups, filling them about 3/4 full.
6. Bake for 16-18 minutes, until a toothpick inserted in the center comes out clean. Allow the cupcakes to cool in the pan for 5 minutes, then transfer to a wire rack to cool completely.
7. Make the frosting: In a medium bowl, beat the cream cheese, powdered erythritol, and vanilla extract until smooth and creamy. Add 1-2 tablespoons of almond milk if the frosting is too thick.
8. Frost the cooled cupcakes and serve.

These low-sugar red velvet cupcakes are a healthier take on the classic dessert. The use of applesauce and zero-calorie sweeteners keeps the sugar content low, while the cream cheese frosting provides a rich, indulgent topping.

# Chapter 7 : Desserts

**Baked Apple Slices with Cinnamon**

Prep Time: 10 minutes
Cook Time: 25 minutes
Total Time: 35 minutes
Serves: 4

**Ingredients:**
- 3 medium apples, cored and sliced into 1/4-inch thick rounds
- 1 tablespoon unsalted butter, melted
- 2 tablespoons brown sugar
- 1 teaspoon ground cinnamon
- 1/4 teaspoon ground nutmeg
- Pinch of salt

**Instructions:**
1. Preheat oven to 375°F. Line a baking sheet with parchment paper.
2. Arrange the apple slices in a single layer on the prepared baking sheet.
3. In a small bowl, mix together the melted butter, brown sugar, cinnamon, nutmeg, and salt.
4. Drizzle the cinnamon-sugar mixture evenly over the apple slices, making sure to coat both sides.
5. Bake for 20-25 minutes, flipping the slices halfway through, until the apples are tender and the edges are lightly browned.
6. Serve the baked apple slices warm, either on their own or with a scoop of vanilla ice cream or a drizzle of caramel sauce.

Nutrition Facts (per serving):
Calories: 100
Total Fat: 3g
Saturated Fat: 2g
Cholesterol: 8mg
Sodium: 35mg
Total Carbohydrates: 19g
Fiber: 3g
Sugars: 14g
Protein: 0g

These baked apple slices make a simple and delicious healthy dessert or snack. The cinnamon and brown sugar add warmth and sweetness, while keeping the sugar content relatively low. Enjoy them on their own or pair them with your favorite toppings.

**Black-Eyed Pea Salad**

Prep Time: 15 minutes
Total Time: 15 minutes
Serves: 4

**Ingredients**:
- 1 (15 oz) can black-eyed peas, drained and rinsed
- 1 cup diced cucumber
- 1/2 cup diced red onion
- 1/2 cup diced bell pepper (any color)
- 1/4 cup chopped fresh parsley
- 2 tablespoons olive oil
- 2 tablespoons red wine vinegar
- 1 tablespoon Dijon mustard
- 1 garlic clove, minced
- 1/2 teaspoon salt
- 1/4 teaspoon black pepper

**Instructions:**
1. In a large bowl, combine the drained and rinsed black-eyed peas, diced cucumber, red onion, bell pepper, and chopped parsley.
2. In a small bowl, whisk together the olive oil, red wine vinegar, Dijon mustard, minced garlic, salt, and black pepper.
3. Pour the dressing over the black-eyed pea mixture and toss gently to coat.
4. Cover and refrigerate for at least 30 minutes to allow the flavors to meld.
5. Serve chilled or at room temperature.

Nutrition Facts (per serving):
Calories: 150
Total Fat: 7g
Saturated Fat: 1g
Cholesterol: 0mg
Sodium: 400mg
Total Carbohydrates: 17g
Fiber: 5g
Sugars: 3g
Protein: 6g

This refreshing black-eyed pea salad is a great side dish or light meal. The combination of the protein-rich black-eyed peas, crisp vegetables, and tangy vinaigrette makes it a flavorful and nutritious option. It's perfect for picnics, potlucks, or as a healthy lunch.

**BBQ Tofu with Collard Greens**

Prep Time: 20 minutes
Cook Time: 30 minutes
Total Time: 50 minutes
Serves: 4

**Ingredients:**
Tofu:
- 1 block (14 oz) extra-firm tofu, pressed and cubed
- 1/2 cup barbecue sauce

***Collard Greens:***
- 1 bunch collard greens, stems removed and leaves chopped
- 1 tablespoon olive oil
- 1 onion, diced
- 2 cloves garlic, minced
- 1/4 cup vegetable broth
- 1 tablespoon apple cider vinegar
- 1/4 teaspoon red pepper flakes (optional)
- Salt and pepper to taste

**Instructions:**
1. Preheat oven to 400°F. Line a baking sheet with parchment paper.
2. In a bowl, toss the cubed tofu with the barbecue sauce until evenly coated. Spread the tofu on the prepared baking sheet and bake for 20-25 minutes, flipping halfway, until crispy.
3. While the tofu is baking, heat the olive oil in a large skillet over medium heat. Add the onion and sauté for 3-4 minutes until translucent.
4. Add the garlic and collard greens to the skillet. Pour in the vegetable broth and apple cider vinegar. Season with red pepper flakes (if using), salt, and pepper.
5. Cook the collard greens for 10-15 minutes, stirring occasionally, until tender.
6. Serve the BBQ tofu over the sautéed collard greens.

Nutrition Facts (per serving):
Calories: 220
Total Fat: 10g
Saturated Fat: 1g
Cholesterol: 0mg
Sodium: 580mg
Total Carbohydrates: 20g
Fiber: 5g
Sugars: 10g
Protein: 16g

**Vegetarian Gumbo**

Prep Time: 20 minutes
Cook Time: 45 minutes
Total Time: 1 hour 5 minutes
Serves: 6

**Ingredients**:
- 2 tablespoons olive oil
- 1 onion, diced
- 1 bell pepper, diced
- 3 celery stalks, diced
- 3 garlic cloves, minced
- 1/4 cup all-purpose flour
- 4 cups vegetable broth
- 1 (14 oz) can diced tomatoes
- 1 (15 oz) can kidney beans, drained and rinsed
- 1 (15 oz) can chickpeas, drained and rinsed
- 1 cup sliced okra (fresh or frozen)
- 1 bay leaf
- 1 teaspoon smoked paprika
- 1 teaspoon dried thyme
- 1/2 teaspoon cayenne pepper (or to taste)
- Salt and black pepper to taste
- Cooked rice, for serving

**Instructions**:

1. In a large pot or Dutch oven, heat the olive oil over medium heat. Add the onion, bell pepper, celery, and garlic. Sauté for 5-7 minutes until the vegetables are softened.

2. Sprinkle the flour over the vegetables and stir to coat. Cook for 2-3 minutes, stirring constantly, to make a roux.

3. Gradually whisk in the vegetable broth, scraping up any browned bits from the bottom of the pot. Bring the mixture to a simmer.

4. Add the diced tomatoes, kidney beans, chickpeas, okra, bay leaf, smoked paprika, thyme, and cayenne. Season with salt and black pepper to taste.

5. Reduce heat to medium-low and let the gumbo simmer for 30-40 minutes, stirring occasionally, until thickened. Remove the bay leaf. Serve the gumbo over cooked rice.

**Nutrition Facts (per serving):**
Calories: 280
Total Fat: 7g
Saturated Fat: 1g
Cholesterol: 0mg
Sodium: 680mg
Total Carbohydrates: 44g
Fiber: 10g
Sugars: 7g
Protein: 11g

This vegetarian gumbo is a hearty and flavorful meatless main dish. The combination of vegetables, beans, and spices creates a rich and satisfying stew-like dish. Serve it over rice for a complete and nutritious meal.

**Sweet Potato and Black Bean Tacos**

Prep Time: 20 minutes
Cook Time: 25 minutes
Total Time: 45 minutes
Serves: 4 (12 tacos)

**Ingredients:**
- 2 medium sweet potatoes, peeled and diced
- 1 tablespoon olive oil
- 1 teaspoon chili powder
- 1/2 teaspoon ground cumin
- 1/4 teaspoon salt
- 1 (15 oz) can black beans, drained and rinsed
- 1/2 cup salsa
- 12 small corn tortillas, warmed
- Toppings: shredded cabbage, diced avocado, chopped cilantro, lime wedges

**Instructions:**
1. Preheat oven to 400°F. Line a baking sheet with parchment paper.
2. In a large bowl, toss the diced sweet potatoes with the olive oil, chili powder, cumin, and salt until evenly coated.
3. Spread the sweet potatoes in a single layer on the prepared baking sheet. Roast for 20-25 minutes, stirring halfway, until tender and lightly browned.
4. In a medium bowl, mash the black beans with a fork or potato masher. Stir in the salsa.
5. To assemble the tacos, place a spoonful of the sweet potato mixture and a spoonful of the black bean mixture into each warm corn tortilla. Top the tacos with shredded cabbage, diced avocado, chopped cilantro, and a squeeze of lime juice.

**Nutrition Facts (per taco):**
Calories: 180
Total Fat: 5g
Saturated Fat: 1g
Cholesterol: 0mg
Sodium: 320mg
Total Carbohydrates: 29g
Fiber: 6g
Sugars: 3g
Protein: 5g

These sweet potato and black bean tacos are a delicious and nutritious vegetarian meal. The roasted sweet potatoes and seasoned black beans provide a flavorful and filling base, while the fresh toppings add crunch and brightness. Enjoy these tacos for a quick and easy weeknight dinner.

**Okra and Tomato Stew**

Prep Time: 15 minutes
Cook Time: 30 minutes
Total Time: 45 minutes
Serves: 4

**Ingredients**:
- 1 lb fresh okra, trimmed and sliced into 1-inch pieces
- 2 tablespoons olive oil
- 1 onion, diced
- 3 cloves garlic, minced
- 1 (14.5 oz) can diced tomatoes
- 1 cup vegetable broth
- 1 teaspoon ground cumin
- 1/2 teaspoon smoked paprika
- 1/4 teaspoon cayenne pepper (or to taste)
- Salt and black pepper to taste
- Chopped fresh parsley for garnish

**Instructions**:
1. In a large skillet or Dutch oven, heat the olive oil over medium heat. Add the sliced okra and sauté for 5-7 minutes, stirring occasionally, until the okra is lightly browned.
2. Add the diced onion and minced garlic to the skillet. Cook for 2-3 minutes, until the onion is translucent.
3. Pour in the diced tomatoes with their juices and the vegetable broth. Stir in the cumin, smoked paprika, and cayenne pepper.
4. Bring the stew to a simmer and let it cook for 20-25 minutes, stirring occasionally, until the okra is very tender.
5. Season the stew with salt and black pepper to taste.
6. Serve the okra and tomato stew warm, garnished with chopped fresh parsley.

Nutrition Facts (per serving):
Calories: 120
Total Fat: 6g
Saturated Fat: 1g
Cholesterol: 0mg
Sodium: 320mg
Total Carbohydrates: 15g
Fiber: 5g
Sugars: 6g
Protein: 3g

**Vegan Jambalaya**

Prep Time: 20 minutes
Cook Time: 40 minutes
Total Time: 1 hour
Serves: 6

**Ingredients:**
- 1 cup uncooked long-grain brown rice
- 2 tablespoons olive oil
- 1 onion, diced
- 1 bell pepper, diced
- 3 celery stalks, diced
- 3 garlic cloves, minced
- 1 (14 oz) can diced tomatoes
- 1 (15 oz) can kidney beans, drained and rinsed
- 1 (15 oz) can chickpeas, drained and rinsed
- 1 cup sliced okra (fresh or frozen)
- 2 cups vegetable broth
- 1 teaspoon smoked paprika
- 1 teaspoon dried thyme
- 1/2 teaspoon cayenne pepper (or to taste)
- 1/2 teaspoon dried oregano
- Salt and black pepper to taste
- Chopped parsley for garnish

**Instructions:**
1. Cook the brown rice according to package instructions. Set aside.

2. In a large pot or Dutch oven, heat the olive oil over medium heat. Add the onion, bell pepper, celery, and garlic. Sauté for 5-7 minutes until the vegetables are softened.

3. Stir in the diced tomatoes, kidney beans, chickpeas, okra, vegetable broth, smoked paprika, thyme, cayenne, and oregano. Season with salt and black pepper to taste.

4. Bring the mixture to a simmer and let it cook for 25-30 minutes, stirring occasionally, until the vegetables are tender and the flavors have melded.

5. Stir the cooked brown rice into the jambalaya.. Serve the vegan jambalaya warm, garnished with chopped parsley.

This vegan jambalaya is a hearty and flavorful plant-based take on the classic Creole dish. The combination of brown rice, vegetables, beans, and Cajun-inspired spices creates a satisfying and nutritious meal. Adjust the spice level to your preference.

**Grilled Portobello Mushrooms**

Prep Time: 10 minutes
Cook Time: 10 minutes
Total Time: 20 minutes
Serves: 4

**Ingredients**:
- 4 large portobello mushroom caps, stems removed
- 2 tablespoons olive oil
- 2 tablespoons balsamic vinegar
- 2 garlic cloves, minced
- 1 teaspoon dried thyme
- 1/2 teaspoon salt
- 1/4 teaspoon black pepper

**Instructions:**
1. Preheat grill or grill pan to medium-high heat.

2. In a shallow dish, whisk together the olive oil, balsamic vinegar, garlic, thyme, salt, and pepper.

3. Add the portobello mushroom caps to the dish and turn to coat both sides evenly with the marinade.

4. Grill the mushrooms for 4-5 minutes per side, or until they are tender and have grill marks.

5. Transfer the grilled portobello mushrooms to a serving plate. Serve the grilled portobellos warm, either on their own or as part of a larger meal, such as on top of a salad or as a burger patty substitute.

Nutrition Facts (per serving):
Calories: 90
Total Fat: 6g
Saturated Fat: 1g
Cholesterol: 0mg
Sodium: 320mg
Total Carbohydrates: 8g
Fiber: 2g
Sugars: 4g
Protein: 3g

These grilled portobello mushrooms make a delicious and versatile vegetarian main dish or side. The balsamic marinade adds a rich, tangy flavor that complements the meaty texture of the mushrooms. Grill them up for a quick and easy meal.

# Chapter 9 : Vegan

**Vegan Mac and Cheese**

**Ingredients:**
- 8 oz elbow macaroni or other small pasta shape
- 1 cup raw cashews, soaked in water for at least 4 hours or overnight
- 1 cup unsweetened almond milk
- 1/2 cup nutritional yeast
- 2 tbsp lemon juice
- 1 tsp Dijon mustard
- 1 tsp garlic powder
- 1 tsp onion powder
- 1/2 tsp salt
- 1/4 tsp ground black pepper

**Instructions:**

1. Cook the pasta according to package instructions. Drain and set aside.

2. Drain and rinse the soaked cashews. Add them to a high-speed blender along with the almond milk, nutritional yeast, lemon juice, mustard, garlic powder, onion powder, salt, and pepper. Blend until completely smooth and creamy.

3. In a large saucepan, combine the cooked pasta and the cashew cheese sauce. Heat over medium, stirring frequently, until the sauce thickens and the pasta is heated through, about 5 minutes.

4. Serve hot, garnished with chopped parsley, chives, or other toppings if desired. Enjoy!

The cashews provide a creamy, cheese-like texture while the nutritional yeast adds a savory, umami flavor. This vegan mac and cheese is sure to satisfy your comfort food cravings!

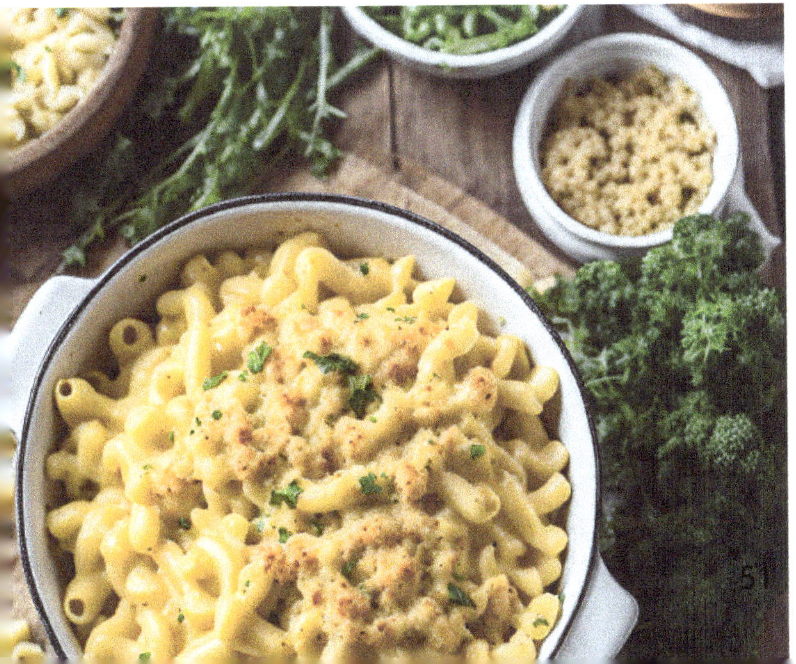

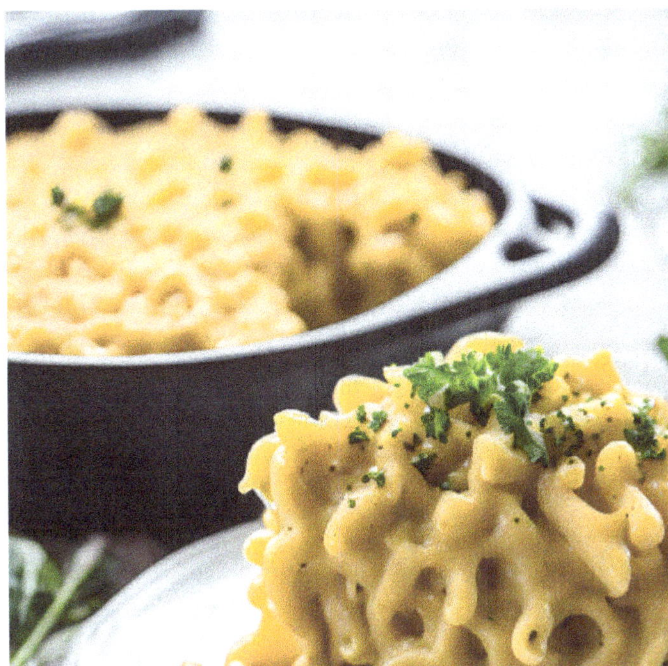

# Chapter 9 : Vegan

**Smoky Tempeh and Collard Greens**

**Ingredients**:
- 8 oz tempeh, cut into 1-inch cubes
- 2 tbsp olive oil
- 1 tsp smoked paprika
- 1/2 tsp garlic powder
- 1/4 tsp cayenne pepper
- Salt and pepper to taste
- 1 bunch collard greens, stems removed and leaves chopped
- 1 cup vegetable broth
- 2 tbsp apple cider vinegar
- 1 tbsp maple syrup

**Instructions:**

1. In a large skillet, heat the olive oil over medium heat. Add the tempeh cubes and sprinkle with the smoked paprika, garlic powder, cayenne, salt, and pepper. Cook, stirring occasionally, until the tempeh is lightly browned on all sides, about 8-10 minutes.

2. Add the chopped collard greens to the skillet and pour in the vegetable broth. Bring to a simmer, then reduce heat to medium-low and cook, stirring occasionally, until the greens are tender, about 10-15 minutes.

3. Stir in the apple cider vinegar and maple syrup. Taste and adjust seasoning as needed.

4. Serve the smoky tempeh and collard greens warm, over rice or quinoa if desired. Enjoy!

The smoky, spiced tempeh pairs perfectly with the tender collard greens in this flavorful and nutritious vegan dish. The apple cider vinegar and maple syrup add a nice balance of acidity and sweetness.

# Chapter 9 : Vegan

**Lentil and Vegetable Stew**

**Ingredients**:
- 1 tbsp olive oil
- 1 onion, diced
- 3 cloves garlic, minced
- 2 carrots, peeled and diced
- 2 celery stalks, diced
- 1 cup brown or green lentils, rinsed
- 4 cups vegetable broth
- 1 (14.5 oz) can diced tomatoes
- 2 tsp dried thyme
- 1 tsp dried oregano
- 1 bay leaf
- Salt and pepper to taste
- 2 cups chopped kale or spinach
- 1/4 cup chopped fresh parsley

**Instructions**:

1. In a large pot or Dutch oven, heat the olive oil over medium heat. Add the onion and sauté for 5 minutes until translucent.

2. Add the garlic, carrots, and celery. Cook for 3-4 minutes, stirring frequently, until the vegetables start to soften.

3. Stir in the lentils, vegetable broth, diced tomatoes, thyme, oregano, and bay leaf. Season with salt and pepper.

4. Bring the stew to a boil, then reduce heat and simmer for 20-25 minutes, until the lentils are tender.

5. Remove the bay leaf. Stir in the chopped kale or spinach and cook for 2-3 minutes until wilted.

6. Remove from heat and stir in the fresh parsley. Taste and adjust seasoning as needed.

7. Serve the lentil and vegetable stew hot, with crusty bread or over cooked grains like quinoa or brown rice.

This hearty, protein-packed stew is full of nutritious vegetables and lentils. It's a comforting and satisfying vegan meal.

# Chapter 9 : Vegan

**Spicy Roasted Cauliflower**

**Ingredients**:
- 1 head of cauliflower, cut into florets
- 2 tbsp olive oil
- 2 tsp chili powder
- 1 tsp smoked paprika
- 1/2 tsp garlic powder
- 1/4 tsp cayenne pepper (or more to taste)
- 1/2 tsp salt
- 1/4 tsp black pepper

**Instructions:**

1. Preheat your oven to 400°F (200°C).

2. In a large bowl, toss the cauliflower florets with the olive oil, chili powder, smoked paprika, garlic powder, cayenne pepper, salt, and black pepper until the cauliflower is evenly coated.

3. Spread the seasoned cauliflower florets in a single layer on a large baking sheet lined with parchment paper.

4. Roast the cauliflower in the preheated oven for 20-25 minutes, flipping halfway through, until the cauliflower is tender and lightly browned.

5. Remove the roasted cauliflower from the oven and serve hot. Garnish with chopped fresh parsley or cilantro if desired.

The combination of chili powder, smoked paprika, and cayenne pepper gives this roasted cauliflower a delicious spicy kick. The high-heat roasting caramelizes the edges of the cauliflower, creating a crispy, flavorful texture.

This spicy roasted cauliflower makes a great side dish or can be enjoyed as a snack. It's a simple and versatile vegan recipe that's sure to please.

# Chapter 9 : Vegan

**Vegan Sweet Potato Pie**

Crust:
- 1 1/4 cups all-purpose flour
- 1/2 tsp salt
- 1/3 cup cold vegan butter or coconut oil
- 3-4 tbsp ice water

Filling:
- 2 cups mashed cooked sweet potatoes (about 2 medium sweet potatoes)
- 1 cup unsweetened almond milk
- 3/4 cup brown sugar
- 1/4 cup maple syrup
- 2 tsp ground cinnamon
- 1 tsp ground ginger
- 1/2 tsp ground nutmeg
- 1/4 tsp ground cloves
- 1/4 tsp salt

**Instructions:**

For the Crust:
1. In a food processor, pulse the flour and salt together. Add the cold vegan butter and pulse until the mixture resembles coarse crumbs.
2. Add the ice water 1 tbsp at a time, pulsing after each addition, until the dough just begins to hold together.
3. Turn the dough out onto a lightly floured surface and shape into a disc. Wrap in plastic and refrigerate for at least 30 minutes.

For the Filling:
1. Preheat oven to 375°F (190°C).
2. In a large bowl, whisk together the mashed sweet potatoes, almond milk, brown sugar, maple syrup, cinnamon, ginger, nutmeg, cloves, and salt until well combined.

Assembly:
1. On a lightly floured surface, roll out the chilled pie dough into a 12-inch circle. Transfer to a 9-inch pie plate.
2. Pour the sweet potato filling into the prepared pie crust.
3. Bake for 45-55 minutes, until the center is set. Allow to cool completely before slicing.

Serve chilled or at room temperature. Top with whipped coconut cream or a sprinkle of cinnamon if desired. Enjoy! This vegan sweet potato pie is rich, creamy, and full of warm spices. It's the perfect plant-based twist on a classic holiday dessert.

# Chapter 9 : Vegan

**Chickpea Salad Sandwich**

**Ingredients**:
- 1 (15 oz) can chickpeas, drained and rinsed
- 1/4 cup vegan mayonnaise (or regular mayonnaise if not vegan)
- 2 tbsp Dijon mustard
- 1 tbsp lemon juice
- 1/4 cup diced celery
- 2 tbsp diced red onion
- 2 tbsp chopped fresh parsley
- 1/4 tsp salt
- 1/4 tsp black pepper

For Serving:
- 8 slices of your favorite bread or rolls
- Lettuce, tomato, sprouts (optional toppings)

**Instructions:**

1. In a medium bowl, use a fork or potato masher to roughly mash the chickpeas, leaving some whole pieces.

2. Add the vegan mayonnaise, Dijon mustard, lemon juice, celery, red onion, parsley, salt, and pepper. Stir everything together until well combined.

3. Taste and adjust any seasonings as needed.

4. To assemble the sandwiches, spread the chickpea salad evenly onto 4 slices of bread. Top with lettuce, tomato, sprouts, or any other desired toppings.

5. Place the remaining 4 slices of bread on top to create 4 complete sandwiches.

6. Serve immediately or refrigerate until ready to eat. The chickpea salad will keep in the fridge for 3-4 days.

This chickpea salad makes a delicious, protein-packed filling for sandwiches. It has a creamy texture and tangy flavor that's perfect for a quick and satisfying plant-based lunch. Enjoy!

# Chapter 9 : Vegan

**Baked Tofu with Spicy Mustard Glaze**

**Ingredients:**
- 1 block (14 oz) extra-firm tofu, pressed and cut into 1-inch cubes
- 2 tbsp olive oil
- 2 tbsp Dijon mustard
- 2 tbsp maple syrup
- 1 tbsp soy sauce or tamari
- 1 tsp sriracha or other hot sauce
- 1/4 tsp garlic powder
- 1/4 tsp ground ginger
- Salt and pepper to taste

**Instructions**:

1. Preheat your oven to 400°F (200°C). Line a baking sheet with parchment paper.

2. In a medium bowl, whisk together the olive oil, Dijon mustard, maple syrup, soy sauce, sriracha, garlic powder, and ground ginger until well combined.

3. Add the tofu cubes to the bowl and gently toss to coat them evenly with the spicy mustard glaze.

4. Arrange the glazed tofu cubes in a single layer on the prepared baking sheet.

5. Bake for 20-25 minutes, flipping the tofu halfway through, until the tofu is crispy and caramelized on the edges.

6. Remove the baked tofu from the oven and season with salt and pepper to taste.

7. Serve the spicy mustard glazed tofu warm, over rice, quinoa, or your favorite salad. Enjoy!

The combination of the Dijon mustard, maple syrup, and sriracha creates a delicious sweet and spicy glaze that coats the crispy baked tofu. This recipe is a great way to add flavor and protein to your meals.

# Chapter 10 : Beverages

**Low-Sugar Lemonade**

**Ingredients:**
- 6 cups water
- 1/2 cup freshly squeezed lemon juice (about 4-6 lemons)
- 2-3 tbsp honey or maple syrup (to taste)
- 1 tsp lemon zest (optional)
- Ice cubes

**Instructions**:

1. In a large pitcher, combine the water and freshly squeezed lemon juice. Stir well.

2. Start by adding 2 tablespoons of honey or maple syrup and stir to dissolve. Taste and add more sweetener if desired, up to 3 tablespoons total.

3. If using, stir in the lemon zest.

4. Fill glasses with ice cubes and pour the lemonade over the ice.

5. Serve immediately and enjoy!

Tips:
- Use fresh, ripe lemons for the best flavor.
- Start with less sweetener and add more to taste. The amount needed will depend on the tartness of your lemons.
- For a fizzy twist, top off the lemonade with some sparkling water or club soda.
- Garnish with lemon slices or mint leaves.

This low-sugar lemonade is a healthier alternative to store-bought versions, which can be high in added sugars. The natural sweetness from the honey or maple syrup complements the tart lemon perfectly. Enjoy this refreshing drink on a hot day!

# Chapter 10 : Beverages



**Green Smoothie**

**Ingredients:**
- 1 cup unsweetened almond milk (or other non-dairy milk)
- 1 cup packed baby spinach or kale
- 1 ripe banana, frozen
- 1/2 cup frozen pineapple chunks
- 1 tbsp chia seeds or ground flaxseeds
- 1 tsp honey or maple syrup (optional)

**Instructions:**

1. Add the almond milk, spinach/kale, banana, pineapple, and chia/flax seeds to a high-speed blender.

2. Blend on high speed until the mixture is smooth and creamy, about 1-2 minutes.

3. Taste and add honey or maple syrup if you'd like it a bit sweeter.

4. Pour the green smoothie into a glass and enjoy immediately.

Tips:
- Use frozen fruit for a thicker, colder smoothie.
- Adjust the amount of milk to reach your desired consistency.
- Try adding other greens like kale, swiss chard, or collard greens.
- Experiment with different fruit combinations like mango, berries, or apple.
- Add a scoop of protein powder or nut butter for extra nutrition.
- Garnish with a sprinkle of cinnamon, shredded coconut, or a slice of lemon.

This green smoothie is packed with vitamins, minerals, and fiber from the leafy greens and fruit. It's a great way to start your day or have as a healthy snack. Enjoy the refreshing, nutrient-dense blend!

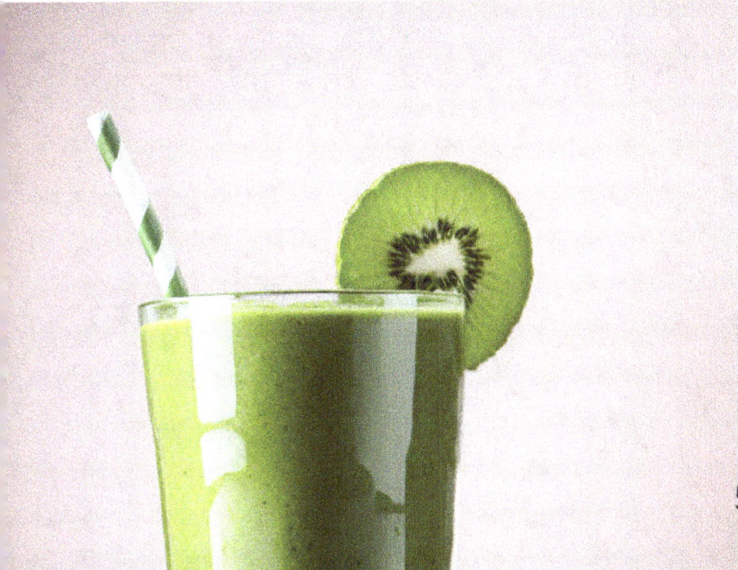
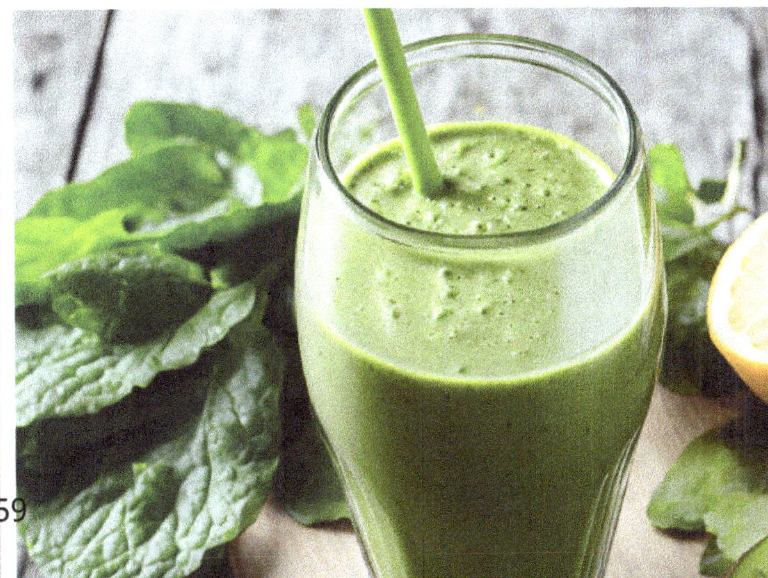

# Chapter 10 : Beverages

**Hibiscus Iced Tea**

**Ingredients**:
- 6 cups water
- 1/2 cup dried hibiscus flowers (or 6 hibiscus tea bags)
- 1/4 cup honey or agave nectar (or to taste)
- 1 tbsp fresh lemon juice
- Lemon slices for garnish (optional)

**Instructions**:

1. In a medium saucepan, bring the 6 cups of water to a boil.

2. Remove the pan from heat and add the dried hibiscus flowers (or tea bags). Let steep for 10-15 minutes.

3. Strain the tea through a fine mesh sieve to remove the hibiscus flowers. Discard the flowers.

4. Stir in the honey or agave nectar until dissolved. Start with 1/4 cup and add more to taste if desired.

5. Stir in the fresh lemon juice.

6. Allow the tea to cool to room temperature, then refrigerate for at least 2 hours until chilled.

7. Serve the hibiscus iced tea over ice. Garnish with lemon slices if desired.

Tips:
- For a stronger hibiscus flavor, steep the flowers for 15-20 minutes.
- Adjust the sweetener to your taste preferences.
- You can also add a few sprigs of fresh mint to the tea.
- Freeze the tea in ice cube trays for easy hibiscus ice cubes.

Hibiscus tea is naturally tart and tangy, with a beautiful deep red color. The honey or agave balances the tartness, creating a refreshing and slightly sweet iced tea. Enjoy this vibrant, antioxidant-rich beverage!

# Chapter 10 : Beverages

**Cucumber Mint Water**

**Ingredients:**
- 1 medium cucumber, sliced
- 10-12 fresh mint leaves
- 6 cups cold water
- Ice cubes

**Instructions**:

1. In a large pitcher or beverage dispenser, add the sliced cucumber and fresh mint leaves.

2. Pour the cold water over the cucumber and mint.

3. Stir gently to combine.

4. Refrigerate for at least 2 hours, or up to 8 hours, to allow the flavors to infuse the water.

5. When ready to serve, fill glasses with ice cubes and pour the cucumber mint water over the ice.

Tips:
- For a stronger mint flavor, gently muddle or bruise the mint leaves before adding to the water.
- Try using a combination of cucumber and lemon slices for extra flavor.
- Add a few thin lemon or lime slices for garnish.
- Swap out the mint for other fresh herbs like basil, rosemary, or thyme.
- Refill the pitcher with more water as needed to maintain the flavor.

This cucumber mint water is a refreshing and hydrating infused water that's perfect for hot summer days. The cool, crisp cucumber and fragrant mint create a delightful flavor combination. Enjoy this healthy, low-calorie beverage to stay hydrated!

# Chapter 10 : Beverages

**Peach Iced Tea**

**Ingredients**:
- 6 cups water
- 4 black tea bags
- 1/2 cup fresh peach puree (about 2-3 ripe peaches, peeled and blended)
- 1/4 cup honey or agave nectar (or to taste)
- 1 tbsp lemon juice
- Sliced peaches for garnish (optional)

**Instructions**:

1. In a medium saucepan, bring the 6 cups of water to a boil. Remove from heat and add the 4 black tea bags. Let steep for 5-7 minutes.

2. Remove the tea bags and stir in the peach puree, honey/agave, and lemon juice until well combined.

3. Allow the tea to cool to room temperature, then refrigerate for at least 2 hours until chilled.

4. Fill glasses with ice and pour the peach iced tea over the ice.

5. Garnish with sliced fresh peaches, if desired.

Tips:
- Use ripe, juicy peaches for the best flavor.
- Adjust the amount of honey/agave to your desired sweetness level.
- For a creamier texture, blend 1/2 cup of the iced tea with 1/4 cup of milk or non-dairy milk.
- Try adding a splash of peach schnapps or white rum for an adult version.
- Freeze the tea in ice cube trays for peach-flavored ice cubes.

This refreshing peach iced tea is the perfect summer drink. The natural sweetness of the peaches pairs beautifully with the bold black tea. Enjoy this fruity, thirst-quenching beverage!

# Chapter 10 : Beverages

**Berry Infused Water**

**Ingredients**:
- 1 cup mixed berries (such as raspberries, blackberries, blueberries)
- 1 lemon, sliced
- 8 cups cold water
- Ice cubes

**Instructions:**

1. In a large pitcher or beverage dispenser, add the mixed berries and lemon slices.

2. Pour the cold water over the fruit.

3. Stir gently to combine.

4. Refrigerate for at least 2 hours, or up to 8 hours, to allow the flavors to infuse the water.

5. When ready to serve, fill glasses with ice cubes and pour the berry infused water over the ice.

Tips:
- Try using a combination of different berries like strawberries, blueberries, raspberries, and blackberries.
- Add a few sprigs of fresh mint or basil for an extra flavor boost.
- Swap out the lemon for other citrus fruits like orange or lime slices.
- For a sweeter infusion, muddle the berries slightly before adding the water.
- Refill the pitcher with more water as needed to maintain the flavor.

This berry infused water is a refreshing and healthy alternative to sugary drinks. The natural sweetness and vibrant colors of the berries make it a visually appealing and delicious way to stay hydrated. Enjoy this infused water on a hot day or as a flavorful addition to your daily water intake.

# Chapter 10 : Beverages

**Ginger Turmeric Tea**

Ingredients:
- 4 cups water
- 1-inch piece of fresh ginger, peeled and sliced
- 1 tsp ground turmeric
- 1 tbsp honey (or to taste)
- 1 tbsp lemon juice
- Pinch of black pepper

**Instructions**:

1. In a medium saucepan, bring the 4 cups of water to a boil over high heat.

2. Once boiling, reduce the heat to medium-low and add the sliced ginger. Simmer for 5-7 minutes to allow the ginger to infuse the water.

3. Stir in the ground turmeric and continue simmering for 2-3 more minutes.

4. Remove the pan from the heat and stir in the honey and lemon juice until the honey is fully dissolved.

5. Strain the tea through a fine mesh sieve to remove the ginger slices.

6. Pour the ginger turmeric tea into mugs and garnish with a pinch of black pepper.

7. Serve hot and enjoy!

Tips:
- For a stronger ginger flavor, use a larger piece of fresh ginger.
- Adjust the honey to your desired sweetness level.
- Add a cinnamon stick or a few cloves for extra warmth and flavor.
- Try using fresh turmeric root instead of ground, if available.
- Refrigerate any leftover tea and enjoy it chilled.

This ginger turmeric tea is a comforting and nourishing beverage. The combination of anti-inflammatory ginger and turmeric, along with the touch of honey and lemon, makes it a soothing and healthy drink. Enjoy this tea when you need a warm pick-me-up!

# Chapter 11 : Healthy Fish and Shellfish

**Grilled Salmon with Avocado Salsa**

**Ingredients:**
Salmon:
- 4 (6 oz) salmon fillets
- 2 tbsp olive oil
- 1 tsp chili powder
- 1 tsp garlic powder
- Salt and pepper to taste

Avocado Salsa:
- 1 ripe avocado, diced
- 1 tomato, diced
- 1/4 cup diced red onion
- 2 tbsp chopped fresh cilantro
- 1 tbsp lime juice
- 1 tsp olive oil
- 1/4 tsp salt

**Instructions:**

1. Preheat your grill or grill pan to medium-high heat.

2. In a small bowl, mix together the olive oil, chili powder, garlic powder, salt, and pepper. Rub this seasoning mixture all over the salmon fillets.

3. Grill the salmon for 4-6 minutes per side, or until it flakes easily with a fork and reaches your desired doneness.

4. While the salmon is grilling, prepare the avocado salsa. In a medium bowl, gently combine the diced avocado, tomato, red onion, cilantro, lime juice, olive oil, and salt.

5. Serve the grilled salmon fillets warm, topped with the fresh avocado salsa.

Tips:
- Use ripe, creamy avocados for the best texture in the salsa.
- Adjust the amount of chili powder to control the spice level.
- Garnish with additional cilantro or a squeeze of lime juice.
- Serve with roasted vegetables or a side salad for a complete meal.

The cool, creamy avocado salsa provides a delicious contrast to the smoky, grilled salmon. This healthy and flavorful dish is perfect for a summer meal.

# Chapter 11 : Healthy Fish and Shellfish

**Cajun Shrimp and Grits**

**Ingredients**:
Grits:
- 1 cup quick-cooking grits
- 4 cups vegetable or chicken broth
- 1/2 cup unsweetened almond milk
- 2 tbsp vegan butter or olive oil
- 1/2 tsp salt
- 1/4 tsp black pepper

Shrimp:
- 1 lb large shrimp, peeled and deveined
- 2 tbsp Cajun seasoning
- 2 tbsp olive oil
- 3 cloves garlic, minced
- 1 red bell pepper, diced
- 1 cup diced tomatoes
- 2 tbsp chopped fresh parsley

**Instructions**:

1. In a medium saucepan, bring the broth and almond milk to a boil over high heat. Slowly whisk in the grits and reduce heat to low. Cook, stirring frequently, until the grits are thick and creamy, about 5-7 minutes. Stir in the vegan butter, salt, and pepper. Keep warm.

2. In a large skillet, toss the shrimp with the Cajun seasoning until evenly coated.

3. Heat the olive oil in the skillet over medium-high heat. Add the seasoned shrimp and sauté for 2-3 minutes per side, until opaque and cooked through.

4. Add the minced garlic, bell pepper, and diced tomatoes to the skillet. Cook for 2-3 minutes, stirring frequently, until the vegetables are tender.

5. Spoon the creamy grits into serving bowls. Top with the Cajun shrimp and vegetable mixture. Garnish with chopped fresh parsley. Serve hot and enjoy!

Tips:
- Use quick-cooking grits to save time.
- Adjust the amount of Cajun seasoning to your desired spice level.
- Substitute the almond milk with regular dairy milk if preferred.
- Add sliced green onions or crumbled bacon for extra flavor.

# Chapter 11 : Healthy Fish and Shellfish

**Blackened Catfish**

**Ingredients**:
- 4 (6 oz) catfish fillets
- 2 tbsp Cajun or Blackened seasoning
- 2 tbsp olive oil
- 1 tbsp unsalted butter
- Lemon wedges for serving

Cajun Seasoning:
- 2 tsp paprika
- 1 tsp garlic powder
- 1 tsp onion powder
- 1 tsp dried oregano
- 1 tsp dried thyme
- 1/2 tsp cayenne pepper
- 1/2 tsp black pepper
- 1/4 tsp salt

**Instructions:**

1. In a small bowl, mix together all the ingredients for the Cajun seasoning.

2. Pat the catfish fillets dry with paper towels and generously coat both sides with the Cajun seasoning.

3. Heat the olive oil and butter in a large skillet over high heat.

4. When the oil is hot, add the seasoned catfish fillets to the skillet. Cook for 3-4 minutes per side, until the fish is blackened and cooked through.

5. Carefully transfer the blackened catfish to a plate. Serve immediately with lemon wedges.

Tips:
- Use a cast-iron skillet or heavy-duty nonstick pan for best results.
- Make sure the oil is very hot before adding the fish to get that nice blackened crust.
- Adjust the amount of cayenne pepper to control the spice level.
- Serve the blackened catfish with sides like rice, roasted vegetables, or a fresh salad.
- Leftover seasoning can be stored in an airtight container for future use.

The bold Cajun seasoning creates a delicious, crispy crust on the tender catfish fillets. This blackened catfish is packed with flavor and makes for a quick and easy weeknight meal

# Chapter 11 : Healthy Fish and Shellfish

**Baked Tilapia with Herbs**

**Ingredients:**
- 4 (6 oz) tilapia fillets
- 2 tbsp olive oil
- 2 tbsp chopped fresh parsley
- 2 tbsp chopped fresh basil
- 1 tbsp chopped fresh thyme
- 2 cloves garlic, minced
- 1 tsp lemon zest
- 1/2 tsp salt
- 1/4 tsp black pepper

**Instructions:**

1. Preheat your oven to 400°F (200°C). Lightly grease a baking dish or line it with parchment paper.

2. In a small bowl, mix together the olive oil, parsley, basil, thyme, garlic, lemon zest, salt, and pepper.

3. Place the tilapia fillets in the prepared baking dish. Spoon the herb mixture evenly over the top of the fish, making sure to coat all the fillets.

4. Bake the tilapia for 15-18 minutes, or until the fish flakes easily with a fork and is opaque throughout.

5. Serve the baked tilapia with herbs immediately, garnished with additional fresh herbs if desired.

Tips:
- Use a combination of your favorite fresh herbs, such as dill, cilantro, or oregano.
- Adjust the amount of garlic and lemon zest to your taste preferences.
- For extra flavor, you can add a squeeze of fresh lemon juice over the fish before serving.
- Serve the baked tilapia with roasted vegetables, a fresh salad, or steamed rice for a complete meal.
- Leftovers can be refrigerated for up to 3 days and reheated gently in the oven or microwave.

This baked tilapia with herbs is a simple, yet flavorful way to prepare this mild, versatile fish. The fresh herbs and lemon zest add a bright, aromatic touch to the tender, flaky tilapia.

# Chapter 11 : Healthy Fish and Shellfish

**Seafood Gumbo**

**Ingredients:**
- 1/2 cup all-purpose flour
- 1/2 cup vegetable oil
- 1 large onion, diced
- 1 green bell pepper, diced
- 3 celery stalks, diced
- 4 cloves garlic, minced
- 1 lb peeled and deveined shrimp
- 1 lb lump crabmeat, picked over for shells
- 1 lb crawfish tails, peeled (or substitute more shrimp)
- 6 cups seafood or chicken broth
- 1 (14.5 oz) can diced tomatoes
- 2 bay leaves
- 1 tsp dried thyme
- 1 tsp dried oregano
- 1/2 tsp cayenne pepper
- 1/2 tsp smoked paprika
- Salt and black pepper to taste
- Cooked white rice, for serving

**Instructions:**

1. In a large heavy-bottomed pot or Dutch oven, make a roux by whisking together the flour and vegetable oil over medium heat. Cook, stirring constantly, until the roux is a dark caramel color, about 15-20 minutes.

2. Add the diced onion, bell pepper, celery, and garlic to the pot. Cook for 5-7 minutes, stirring frequently, until the vegetables are softened.

3. Stir in the shrimp, crabmeat, and crawfish (or additional shrimp). Cook for 2-3 minutes, just until the seafood starts to turn opaque.

4. Pour in the seafood or chicken broth and add the diced tomatoes, bay leaves, thyme, oregano, cayenne, and smoked paprika. Season with salt and black pepper to taste.

5. Bring the gumbo to a boil, then reduce the heat and let it simmer for 30-45 minutes, stirring occasionally, until the flavors have melded and the gumbo has thickened.

6. Serve the seafood gumbo hot, over cooked white rice. Garnish with chopped green onions or parsley, if desired.

# Chapter 11 : Healthy Fish and Shellfish

**Lemon Garlic Shrimp**

**Ingredients:**
- 1 lb large shrimp, peeled and deveined
- 3 tbsp olive oil
- 4 cloves garlic, minced
- 1/4 cup freshly squeezed lemon juice (about 2 lemons)
- 2 tbsp chopped fresh parsley
- 1/4 tsp red pepper flakes (optional)
- Salt and black pepper to taste
- Lemon wedges for serving

**Instructions**:

1. In a large skillet, heat the olive oil over medium-high heat.

2. Add the minced garlic and cook for 1 minute, stirring constantly, until fragrant.

3. Add the shrimp to the skillet and season with a pinch of salt and black pepper. Cook for 2-3 minutes per side, until the shrimp are opaque and cooked through.

4. Stir in the freshly squeezed lemon juice and chopped parsley. Cook for an additional 1-2 minutes, allowing the flavors to combine.

5. If using, sprinkle the red pepper flakes over the shrimp.

6. Taste and adjust seasoning as needed, adding more salt, pepper, or lemon juice to your preference.

7. Serve the lemon garlic shrimp immediately, with lemon wedges on the side.

Tips:
- Use large, fresh shrimp for the best texture and flavor.
- Adjust the amount of red pepper flakes to control the spice level.
- Serve the shrimp over pasta, rice, or with crusty bread to soak up the delicious lemon-garlic sauce.
- For extra flavor, add a splash of white wine or dry vermouth to the skillet.
- Garnish with additional chopped parsley or lemon zest.

This quick and easy lemon garlic shrimp dish is bursting with bright, zesty flavors. It makes a perfect weeknight meal or a simple yet impressive appetizer.

# Chapter 11 : Healthy Fish and Shellfish

**Baked Fish Tacos**

**Ingredients:**
- 1 lb white fish fillets (such as tilapia, cod, or halibut), cut into 1-inch pieces
- 2 tbsp olive oil
- 1 tsp chili powder
- 1 tsp ground cumin
- 1/2 tsp garlic powder
- 1/2 tsp salt
- 8-10 small corn or flour tortillas
- 1 cup shredded cabbage or coleslaw mix
- 1 avocado, diced
- 1/4 cup crumbled queso fresco or feta cheese
- 2 tbsp chopped fresh cilantro
- Lime wedges for serving

Creamy Chipotle Sauce:
- 1/2 cup plain Greek yogurt
- 2 tbsp mayonnaise
- 1 tbsp lime juice
- 1 tsp adobo sauce from canned chipotle peppers
- 1/4 tsp salt

**Instructions**:

1. Preheat your oven to 400°F (200°C). Line a baking sheet with parchment paper.

2. In a medium bowl, toss the fish pieces with the olive oil, chili powder, cumin, garlic powder, and salt until evenly coated.

3. Arrange the seasoned fish pieces in a single layer on the prepared baking sheet. Bake for 12-15 minutes, until the fish is opaque and flakes easily with a fork.

4. While the fish is baking, make the creamy chipotle sauce. In a small bowl, whisk together the Greek yogurt, mayonnaise, lime juice, adobo sauce, and salt.

5. Warm the tortillas according to package instructions.

6. To assemble the tacos, place some of the baked fish pieces in each tortilla. Top with shredded cabbage, diced avocado, crumbled queso fresco, and chopped cilantro.

7. Drizzle the creamy chipotle sauce over the tacos and serve with lime wedges.

**Chicken and Vegetable Stew**

**Ingredients:**
- 1 lb boneless, skinless chicken thighs, cut into 1-inch pieces
- 2 tbsp olive oil
- 1 onion, diced
- 3 carrots, peeled and sliced
- 2 celery stalks, sliced
- 3 cloves garlic, minced
- 1 tsp dried thyme
- 1 tsp dried rosemary
- 1/2 tsp smoked paprika
- 4 cups low-sodium chicken broth
- 1 (14.5 oz) can diced tomatoes
- 2 medium potatoes, peeled and cubed
- 1 cup frozen peas
- Salt and black pepper to taste
- Chopped fresh parsley for garnish

**Instructions:**

1. In a large pot or Dutch oven, heat the olive oil over medium-high heat. Add the chicken and cook for 3-4 minutes, until lightly browned on all sides. Remove the chicken from the pot and set aside.

2. Add the onion, carrots, celery, and garlic to the pot. Sauté for 5-7 minutes, until the vegetables start to soften.

3. Stir in the thyme, rosemary, and smoked paprika. Cook for 1 minute, until fragrant.

4. Pour in the chicken broth and diced tomatoes. Bring the mixture to a boil.

5. Add the cubed potatoes and the cooked chicken back to the pot. Reduce heat to medium-low and simmer for 20-25 minutes, until the potatoes are tender.

6. Stir in the frozen peas and cook for an additional 5 minutes.

7. Season the stew with salt and black pepper to taste.

8. Serve the chicken and vegetable stew hot, garnished with chopped fresh parsley.

This comforting stew is packed with tender chicken, hearty vegetables, and a flavorful broth. It's a perfect one-pot meal for a chilly day. Enjoy!

**Turkey and Sweet Potato Chili**

**Ingredients:**
- 1 lb ground turkey
- 1 tbsp olive oil
- 1 onion, diced
- 3 cloves garlic, minced
- 2 medium sweet potatoes, peeled and cubed
- 1 red bell pepper, diced
- 2 tbsp chili powder
- 1 tsp ground cumin
- 1 tsp dried oregano
- 1/2 tsp smoked paprika
- 1/4 tsp cayenne pepper (or to taste)
- 1 (15 oz) can diced tomatoes
- 1 (15 oz) can black beans, drained and rinsed
- 1 (15 oz) can kidney beans, drained and rinsed
- 2 cups low-sodium chicken or vegetable broth
- Salt and black pepper to taste
- Chopped cilantro, sour cream, and shredded cheese for serving (optional)

**Instructions:**

1. In a large pot or Dutch oven, cook the ground turkey over medium-high heat, breaking it up with a wooden spoon, until browned and cooked through, about 5-7 minutes. Drain any excess fat.

2. Add the olive oil to the pot, then stir in the diced onion and minced garlic. Cook for 2-3 minutes until the onion is translucent.

3. Add the cubed sweet potatoes, diced bell pepper, chili powder, cumin, oregano, smoked paprika, and cayenne pepper. Stir to combine and cook for 2-3 minutes.

4. Pour in the diced tomatoes, black beans, kidney beans, and chicken/vegetable broth. Stir to combine.

5. Bring the chili to a boil, then reduce the heat to medium-low. Simmer for 20-25 minutes, stirring occasionally, until the sweet potatoes are tender.

6. Season the chili with salt and black pepper to taste.

7. Serve the turkey and sweet potato chili hot, topped with chopped cilantro, sour cream, and shredded cheese if desired.

# Chapter 12 : Healthy One-Pot Meals

**Southern Vegetable Soup**

**Ingredients:**
- 2 tbsp olive oil
- 1 onion, diced
- 3 carrots, peeled and sliced
- 3 celery stalks, sliced
- 3 cloves garlic, minced
- 1 lb Yukon Gold potatoes, peeled and cubed
- 1 (15 oz) can diced tomatoes
- 6 cups low-sodium vegetable or chicken broth
- 1 bay leaf
- 1 tsp dried thyme
- 1 tsp dried oregano
- 1/2 tsp smoked paprika
- Salt and black pepper to taste
- 1 cup frozen green beans
- 1 cup frozen corn kernels
- 1 cup frozen peas
- Chopped fresh parsley for garnish

**Instructions**:

1. In a large pot or Dutch oven, heat the olive oil over medium heat. Add the diced onion, sliced carrots, and sliced celery. Sauté for 5-7 minutes, until the vegetables start to soften.

2. Stir in the minced garlic and cook for 1 minute, until fragrant.

3. Add the cubed potatoes, diced tomatoes, vegetable/chicken broth, bay leaf, thyme, oregano, and smoked paprika. Season with salt and black pepper to taste.

4. Bring the soup to a boil, then reduce the heat to medium-low. Simmer for 15-20 minutes, until the potatoes are tender.

5. Stir in the frozen green beans, corn, and peas. Cook for an additional 5-7 minutes, until the vegetables are heated through.

6. Remove the bay leaf. Taste and adjust seasoning as needed.

7. Serve the Southern vegetable soup hot, garnished with chopped fresh parsley.

This hearty, veggie-packed soup is a comforting and satisfying meal. The combination of potatoes, tomatoes, and mixed vegetables makes it a delicious and nutritious dish. Enjoy!

# Chapter 12 : Healthy One-Pot Meals

**One-Pot Cajun Pasta**

**Ingredients**:
- 8 oz penne or other short pasta
- 1 tbsp olive oil
- 1 lb boneless, skinless chicken breasts, cut into 1-inch pieces
- 1 onion, diced
- 3 cloves garlic, minced
- 1 red bell pepper, diced
- 1 tsp Cajun seasoning
- 1/2 tsp smoked paprika
- 1/4 tsp cayenne pepper (or to taste)
- 1 (14.5 oz) can diced tomatoes
- 2 cups low-sodium chicken broth
- 1 cup heavy cream or half-and-half
- 1/2 cup grated Parmesan cheese
- Salt and black pepper to taste
- Chopped fresh parsley for garnish

**Instructions**:

1. In a large pot or Dutch oven, bring salted water to a boil. Add the penne pasta and cook according to package instructions until al dente. Drain and set aside.

2. In the same pot, heat the olive oil over medium-high heat. Add the diced chicken and cook for 3-4 minutes, until lightly browned.

3. Add the diced onion, minced garlic, and diced bell pepper to the pot. Sauté for 5-7 minutes, until the vegetables are softened.

4. Stir in the Cajun seasoning, smoked paprika, and cayenne pepper. Cook for 1 minute, until fragrant.

5. Pour in the diced tomatoes and chicken broth. Bring the mixture to a simmer and let it cook for 5-7 minutes.

6. Reduce the heat to medium-low and stir in the heavy cream or half-and-half. Add the cooked penne pasta and grated Parmesan cheese. Toss to combine.

7. Let the pasta simmer for 2-3 minutes, until the sauce has thickened slightly.

8. Season the Cajun pasta with salt and black pepper to taste. Serve the one-pot Cajun pasta hot, garnished with chopped fresh parsley.

# Chapter 12 : Healthy One-Pot Meals

**Quinoa Jambalaya**

**Ingredients:**
- 1 cup uncooked quinoa, rinsed
- 2 cups low-sodium vegetable or chicken broth
- 1 tbsp olive oil
- 1 onion, diced
- 3 celery stalks, diced
- 1 green bell pepper, diced
- 3 cloves garlic, minced
- 1 lb andouille sausage, sliced (or use a plant-based sausage)
- 1 (14.5 oz) can diced tomatoes
- 1 tsp Cajun or Creole seasoning
- 1/2 tsp smoked paprika
- 1/4 tsp cayenne pepper (or to taste)
- Salt and black pepper to taste
- Chopped green onions and parsley for garnish

**Instructions:**

1. In a medium saucepan, combine the rinsed quinoa and vegetable/chicken broth. Bring to a boil, then reduce heat to low, cover, and simmer for 15-20 minutes, until the quinoa is cooked and the liquid is absorbed. Fluff with a fork and set aside.

2. In a large skillet or Dutch oven, heat the olive oil over medium-high heat. Add the diced onion, celery, and bell pepper. Sauté for 5-7 minutes, until the vegetables are softened.

3. Stir in the minced garlic and sliced andouille sausage. Cook for 2-3 minutes, until the garlic is fragrant and the sausage is lightly browned.

4. Add the diced tomatoes, Cajun/Creole seasoning, smoked paprika, and cayenne pepper. Stir to combine.

5. Gently fold the cooked quinoa into the vegetable and sausage mixture. Season with salt and black pepper to taste.

6. Reduce the heat to low and let the jambalaya simmer for 5-10 minutes, allowing the flavors to meld. Serve the quinoa jambalaya hot, garnished with chopped green onions and parsley.

This quinoa jambalaya is a healthier, protein-packed twist on the classic Cajun dish. The quinoa adds a nutty texture and extra nutrition, while the Cajun spices and andouille sausage provide the signature bold flavors.

# Chapter 12 : Healthy One-Pot Meals

**Beef and Collard Green Stew**

**Ingredients:**
- 1 lb beef stew meat, cut into 1-inch cubes
- 2 tbsp olive oil
- 1 onion, diced
- 3 cloves garlic, minced
- 1 lb collard greens, stems removed and leaves chopped
- 4 cups low-sodium beef broth
- 1 (14.5 oz) can diced tomatoes
- 2 medium potatoes, peeled and cubed
- 1 tsp dried thyme
- 1 tsp smoked paprika
- 1/2 tsp cayenne pepper (or to taste)
- Salt and black pepper to taste
- Chopped fresh parsley for garnish

**Instructions:**

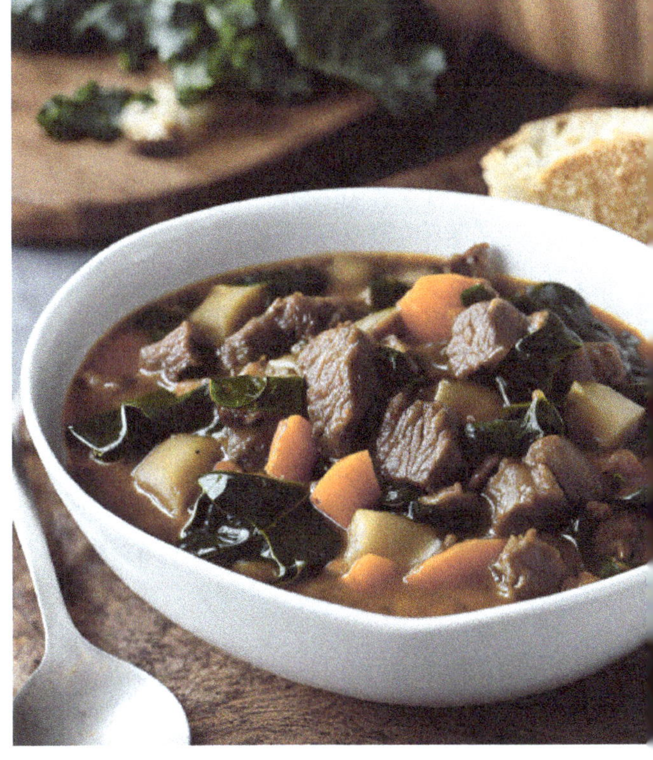

1. In a large pot or Dutch oven, heat the olive oil over medium-high heat. Add the beef cubes and brown on all sides, about 3-4 minutes per side. Remove the beef from the pot and set aside.

2. Reduce the heat to medium and add the diced onion to the pot. Sauté for 5-7 minutes, until the onion is translucent.

3. Stir in the minced garlic and cook for 1 minute, until fragrant.

4. Add the chopped collard greens to the pot and cook for 2-3 minutes, until the greens start to wilt.

5. Pour in the beef broth and diced tomatoes. Bring the mixture to a simmer.

6. Return the browned beef cubes to the pot, along with the cubed potatoes, dried thyme, smoked paprika, and cayenne pepper. Season with salt and black pepper to taste.

7. Reduce the heat to medium-low and let the stew simmer for 45-60 minutes, until the beef and potatoes are tender.

8. Taste and adjust seasoning as needed. Serve the beef and collard green stew hot, garnished with chopped fresh parsley.

This hearty, flavorful stew is a delicious way to enjoy tender beef and nutrient-rich collard greens. The combination of spices and vegetables creates a comforting and satisfying meal.

**Seafood Boil**

**Ingredients:**
- 4 cups water
- 2 cups seafood or chicken broth
- 2 lemons, halved
- 2 bay leaves
- 2 tsp Old Bay seasoning
- 1 tsp salt
- 1 lb small red potatoes, halved
- 4 ears of corn, cut into 2-inch pieces
- 1 lb large shrimp, peeled and deveined
- 1 lb mussels, scrubbed and debearded
- 1 lb crawfish or crab legs (optional)
- Melted butter or lemon wedges for serving

**Instructions**:

1. In a large stockpot, combine the water, broth, lemon halves, bay leaves, Old Bay seasoning, and salt. Bring to a boil over high heat.

2. Add the halved potatoes to the boiling liquid and cook for 10 minutes.

3. Add the corn pieces and continue cooking for 5 more minutes.

4. Add the shrimp, mussels, and crawfish/crab legs (if using) to the pot. Cover and cook for 5-7 minutes, until the shrimp are opaque and the mussels have opened up.

5. Drain the seafood boil mixture into a large colander or serving dish, discarding the bay leaves and lemon halves.

6. Serve the seafood boil immediately, with melted butter or lemon wedges on the side for dipping.

Tips:
- Adjust the cooking times as needed based on the size of the seafood.
- Add other vegetables like onions, garlic, or sausage to the boil.
- Serve the seafood boil with crusty bread, coleslaw, or a simple salad.
- For a spicier version, add extra Old Bay seasoning or cayenne pepper.

This classic seafood boil is a fun and flavorful way to enjoy a variety of fresh seafood. The combination of shrimp, mussels, and optional crawfish or crab makes for a truly indulgent and delicious meal.

# Chapter 13 : Classic Dishes

**Baked Fried Chicken**

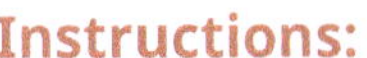

**Ingredients:**
- 8 chicken thighs and/or drumsticks, skin-on and bone-in
- 1 cup buttermilk
- 1 1/2 cups all-purpose flour
- 1 tsp paprika
- 1 tsp garlic powder
- 1 tsp onion powder
- 1 tsp salt
- 1/2 tsp black pepper
- 2 tbsp vegetable oil

**Instructions:**

1. Place the chicken pieces in a large resealable bag or bowl. Pour in the buttermilk and turn the chicken to coat. Cover and refrigerate for at least 30 minutes, up to 24 hours.

2. Preheat your oven to 400°F (200°C). Line a large baking sheet with parchment paper or a silicone baking mat.

3. In a shallow bowl or plate, mix together the flour, paprika, garlic powder, onion powder, salt, and black pepper.

4. Remove the chicken pieces from the buttermilk one at a time, allowing any excess to drip off. Dredge the chicken in the seasoned flour, pressing to help the coating adhere.

5. Place the coated chicken pieces on the prepared baking sheet. Drizzle the vegetable oil over the top of the chicken.

6. Bake for 35-45 minutes, flipping the chicken halfway through, until the skin is golden brown and crispy, and the chicken is cooked through (internal temperature reaches 165°F/75°C). Serve the baked fried chicken hot, garnished with chopped parsley if desired.

Tips:
- For extra crispy skin, broil the chicken for 2-3 minutes at the end of the baking time.
- Use a combination of chicken thighs and drumsticks for a mix of dark and white meat.
- Adjust the baking time as needed based on the size of your chicken pieces.
- Serve the baked fried chicken with mashed potatoes, coleslaw, or biscuits for a classic Southern-style meal.

This baked fried chicken recipe gives you all the flavor and crunch of fried chicken, but with a healthier baked method. The buttermilk and seasoned flour coating create a delicious, crispy exterior.

# Chapter 13 : Classic Dishes

**Southern-style collard greens:**

**Ingredients:**
- 1 lb collard greens, washed and stems removed
- 4 cups chicken or vegetable broth
- 2 tablespoons apple cider vinegar
- 1 tablespoon brown sugar
- 1 teaspoon smoked paprika
- 1/2 teaspoon crushed red pepper flakes (optional for spice)
- 2 cloves garlic, minced
- 1 onion, diced
- 2 tablespoons olive oil
- Salt and pepper to taste

**Instructions:**

1. Rinse the collard greens thoroughly and remove the tough stems. Chop the leaves into 1-inch strips.

2. In a large pot, heat the olive oil over medium heat. Add the onions and sauté for 3-4 minutes until translucent.

3. Add the garlic and sauté for 1 minute until fragrant.

4. Pour in the broth, vinegar, brown sugar, smoked paprika, and red pepper flakes (if using). Bring to a simmer.

5. Add the chopped collard greens to the pot and stir to combine. Cover and let simmer for 45-60 minutes, stirring occasionally, until the greens are very tender.

6. Season with salt and pepper to taste.

7. Serve the collard greens warm, with the cooking liquid spooned over the top. Enjoy!

The long simmering time helps break down the tough collard greens and infuses them with the rich, savory flavors. Feel free to add a splash of hot sauce or a sprinkle of crushed red pepper flakes for extra heat.

# Chapter 13 : Classic Dishes

**Low-Sodium Mac and Cheese**

**Ingredients**:
- 8 oz whole wheat elbow macaroni
- 2 tbsp unsalted butter
- 2 tbsp all-purpose flour
- 2 cups low-fat milk
- 1 cup shredded low-sodium cheddar cheese
- 1/2 cup shredded low-sodium Parmesan cheese
- 1/4 tsp ground black pepper

**Instructions:**

1. Cook the macaroni according to package directions. Drain and set aside.

2. In a medium saucepan, melt the butter over medium heat. Whisk in the flour and cook for 1 minute, stirring constantly.

3. Gradually whisk in the milk and cook, stirring frequently, until the sauce thickens, about 5-7 minutes.

4. Remove the sauce from heat and stir in the cheddar and Parmesan cheeses until melted and smooth.

5. Add the cooked macaroni to the cheese sauce and stir to combine.

6. Season with black pepper.

7. Serve hot.

This recipe uses low-sodium cheese and no added salt to keep the sodium content low. You can also try using whole wheat pasta for added fiber. Enjoy your healthier mac and cheese!

# Chapter 13 : Classic Dishes

**Low-Sodium Cornbread Muffins**

**Ingredients:**
- 1 cup cornmeal
- 1 cup whole wheat flour
- 2 tsp baking powder
- 1/4 tsp baking soda
- 1/4 tsp ground black pepper
- 1 cup low-fat buttermilk
- 1/4 cup unsweetened applesauce
- 2 tbsp honey
- 1 large egg

**Instructions:**

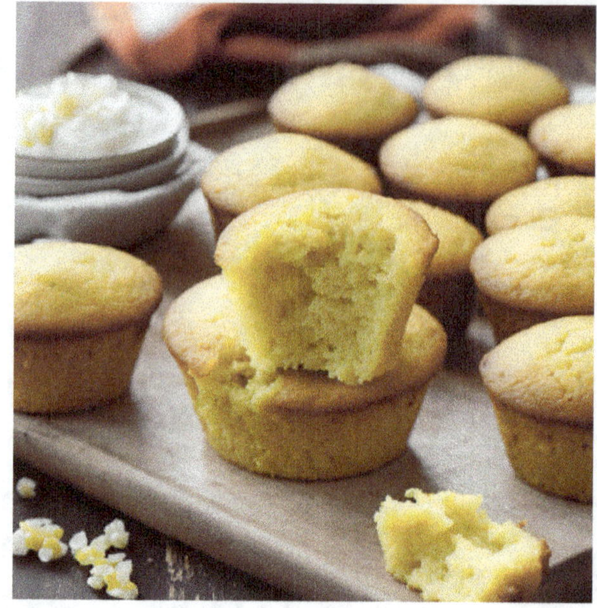

1. Preheat oven to 400°F. Grease a 12-cup muffin tin or line with paper liners.

2. In a large bowl, whisk together the cornmeal, whole wheat flour, baking powder, baking soda, and black pepper.

3. In a separate bowl, whisk together the buttermilk, applesauce, honey, and egg.

4. Pour the wet ingredients into the dry ingredients and stir just until combined (do not overmix).

5. Divide the batter evenly among the prepared muffin cups, filling them about 3/4 full.

6. Bake for 15-18 minutes, until a toothpick inserted in the center comes out clean.

7. Allow the muffins to cool in the pan for 5 minutes before transferring to a wire rack.

These cornbread muffins are low in sodium since they don't contain any added salt. The whole wheat flour and cornmeal provide fiber, and the applesauce and honey add natural sweetness. Enjoy these moist and flavorful muffins!

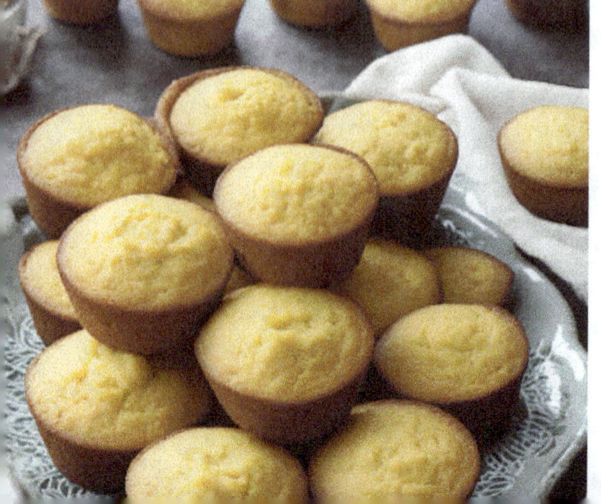

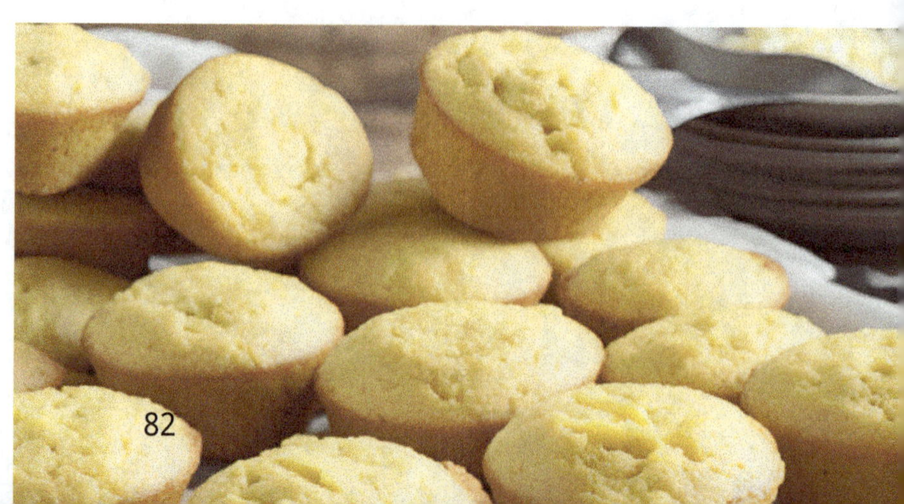

# Chapter 13 : Classic Dishes

**Low-Sodium Hoppin' John**

**Ingredients:**
- 1 cup dried black-eyed peas, soaked overnight and drained
- 4 cups low-sodium vegetable or chicken broth
- 1 bay leaf
- 1 tsp smoked paprika
- 1/2 tsp ground black pepper
- 1 cup cooked brown rice
- 1/2 cup diced onion
- 1/2 cup diced celery
- 1/2 cup diced bell pepper
- 2 cloves garlic, minced
- 2 tbsp chopped fresh parsley

**Instructions:**

1. In a large pot, combine the soaked black-eyed peas, broth, bay leaf, smoked paprika, and black pepper. Bring to a boil.

2. Reduce heat to medium-low, cover, and simmer for 45-60 minutes, until the peas are very tender.

3. Remove the bay leaf. Use a potato masher or the back of a spoon to lightly mash about half of the peas, leaving some whole.

4. Stir in the cooked brown rice, onion, celery, bell pepper, and garlic. Cook for 5-10 minutes, until the vegetables are tender.

5. Remove from heat and stir in the chopped parsley.

6. Serve hot, with additional black pepper to taste.

This low-sodium version of Hoppin' John uses low-sodium broth and omits the traditional ham or bacon, which can be high in sodium. The smoked paprika adds great flavor without the need for salt. Enjoy this healthy and delicious Southern classic!

# Chapter 13 : Classic Dishes

**Low-Sodium Slow Cooker Ribs**

**Ingredients:**
- 2 lbs pork baby back ribs, cut into individual ribs
- 1 cup low-sodium beef or chicken broth
- 1/2 cup no-sugar-added ketchup
- 2 tbsp apple cider vinegar
- 1 tbsp Worcestershire sauce (low-sodium if available)
- 1 tbsp brown sugar
- 1 tsp garlic powder
- 1 tsp onion powder
- 1/2 tsp ground black pepper

**Instructions:**

1. Place the ribs in a slow cooker.

2. In a medium bowl, whisk together the broth, ketchup, vinegar, Worcestershire sauce, brown sugar, garlic powder, onion powder, and black pepper.

3. Pour the sauce mixture over the ribs, making sure they are evenly coated.

4. Cover and cook on low for 7-8 hours, or on high for 4-5 hours, until the ribs are very tender.

5. Remove the ribs from the slow cooker and place them on a baking sheet.

6. Preheat the oven to broil.

7. Broil the ribs for 2-3 minutes per side, until they are lightly charred and caramelized.

8. Serve the ribs hot, with the cooking liquid spooned over the top.

This low-sodium recipe uses a homemade sauce made with low-sodium broth, no-sugar-added ketchup, and minimal added salt. The slow cooking makes the ribs incredibly tender, and the broiling at the end adds a nice caramelized crust. Enjoy these delicious and healthy slow cooker ribs!

# conclucde

**Staying Motivated on a Diabetic Diet**

*Managing diabetes through diet requires commitment, but it doesn't mean sacrificing enjoyment or flavor. By making thoughtful choices and embracing delicious, diabetes-friendly recipes, you can maintain stable blood sugar levels, support heart health, and enhance overall well-being. Here are some tips to stay motivated on your diabetic diet journey:*

1. Celebrate Progress: Recognize and celebrate small victories along the way, whether it's trying a new recipe, reaching a health goal, or making positive changes to your lifestyle.

2. Stay Educated: Continue learning about diabetes management, nutrition, and healthy cooking techniques. Knowledge empowers you to make informed decisions and adapt to new challenges.

3. Build a Support System: Surround yourself with supportive friends, family, or a diabetes support group. Sharing experiences and advice can provide encouragement and motivation.

4. Practice Mindful Eating: Pay attention to hunger cues, portion sizes, and the impact of different foods on your blood sugar levels. Mindful eating promotes enjoyment and helps you make healthier choices.

5. Stay Active: Regular physical activity is essential for managing diabetes. Find activities you enjoy and incorporate them into your daily routine to improve blood sugar control and overall fitness.

**Frequently Asked Questions :** Explore common questions about diabetes management, meal planning, and recipe modifications. Learn from others' experiences and discover practical solutions to everyday challenges.

**Resources for Further Reading :** Discover reputable sources for more information on diabetes, nutrition, and healthy living. From trusted websites to recommended books and publications, expand your knowledge and find additional support.

**Index :** Quickly find recipes, tips, and information throughout the cookbook with a comprehensive index organized by topic and recipe name.

**Acknowledgments :** Recognize the contributions of those who supported the creation of this cookbook, from recipe developers and nutrition experts to friends, family, and the diabetes community.

**Embrace the journey of managing diabetes with positivity and determination. With the recipes and guidance in this cookbook, you have the tools to enjoy delicious soul food while nurturing your health. Here's to vibrant living and savoring every moment on your path to wellness.**

**Tips and Meal Plans for Diabetics**

*Managing diabetes effectively involves thoughtful meal planning and making healthy food choices. Here are some practical tips and meal plans to help you maintain stable blood sugar levels and support overall health:*

**Tips for Diabetics:**

1. Monitor Carbohydrates: Pay attention to the types and amounts of carbohydrates you consume. Focus on whole grains, vegetables, fruits, and legumes, which provide fiber and nutrients while affecting blood sugar more gradually.

2. Choose Lean Proteins: Include lean sources of protein such as poultry, fish, tofu, and legumes in your meals. Protein helps maintain muscle mass and keeps you feeling full.

3. Healthy Fats: Incorporate heart-healthy fats like olive oil, avocados, nuts, and seeds. These fats can improve insulin sensitivity and support cardiovascular health.

4. Portion Control: Be mindful of portion sizes to avoid overeating, which can lead to spikes in blood sugar. Use smaller plates and utensils to help control portions.

5. Stay Hydrated: Drink plenty of water throughout the day to stay hydrated and support kidney function. Limit sugary drinks and opt for water, herbal teas, or flavored water without added sugars.

6. Regular Physical Activity: Engage in regular exercise to help control blood sugar levels, improve insulin sensitivity, and maintain a healthy weight. Aim for at least 150 minutes of moderate-intensity aerobic activity per week.

7. Monitor Blood Sugar Levels: Check your blood sugar levels regularly as recommended by your healthcare provider. This helps you understand how different foods and activities affect your blood sugar.

8. Meal Timing: Try to eat meals and snacks at consistent times each day to help regulate blood sugar levels. Avoid skipping meals, especially breakfast, as it can lead to unstable blood sugar levels.

**Sample Diabetic Meal Plan:**

**Breakfast:**
- Spinach and Mushroom Omelet with Whole Grain Toast
- Fresh Berries
- Herbal Tea or Coffee (unsweetened)

**Mid-Morning Snack:**
- Greek Yogurt with a sprinkle of nuts and seeds

**Lunch:**
- Grilled Chicken Salad with Mixed Greens, Cucumber, Tomato, and Olive Oil Vinaigrette
- Quinoa or Brown Rice (small portion)
- Sparkling Water with Lemon

**Afternoon Snack:**
- Apple slices with a tablespoon of almond butter

**Dinner:**
- Baked Salmon with Lemon and Herbs
- Steamed Broccoli or Asparagus
- Quinoa Pilaf or Cauliflower Rice
- Water or Herbal Tea

**Evening Snack (if needed):**
- Carrot sticks with Hummus

**Additional Tips:**

**- *Meal Prepping:*** Prepare meals and snacks ahead of time to ensure you have healthy options readily available.

**- *Variety:*** Incorporate a variety of foods from different food groups to ensure you get a range of nutrients.

**- *Recipe Modifications:*** Adapt your favorite recipes to be lower in sugar, salt, and unhealthy fats. Experiment with herbs, spices, and natural sweeteners for added flavor.

**- *Consult a Dietitian:*** Consider consulting with a registered dietitian who specializes in diabetes care to personalize meal plans and receive tailored advice.

By following these tips and meal plans, you can effectively manage diabetes while enjoying delicious and nutritious meals that support your overall well-being.

# Here are 20 tips that can help manage diabetes effectively

**Diet and Nutrition**

- 1. Balanced Diet: Focus on a balanced diet with a mix of carbohydrates, proteins, and fats. Choose whole grains over refined grains.

- 2. Portion Control: Keep portion sizes in check to avoid overeating and manage blood sugar levels.

- 3. Low Glycemic Index Foods: Incorporate low glycemic index foods like legumes, whole grains, and non-starchy vegetables.

- 4. Healthy Fats: Include healthy fats from sources like avocados, nuts, seeds, and olive oil.

- 5. Fiber-Rich Foods: Consume fiber-rich foods such as fruits, vegetables, and whole grains to help control blood sugar levels.

- 6. Limit Sugary Foods: Avoid sugary drinks and foods high in sugar. Opt for natural sweeteners like stevia if needed.

- 7. Regular Meals: Eat at regular intervals to maintain steady blood sugar levels.

- 8. Hydration: Stay well-hydrated with water and avoid sugary drinks.

**Exercise**

- 9. Regular Exercise: Aim for at least 150 minutes of moderate-intensity exercise per week, such as brisk walking or cycling.

- 10. Strength Training: Incorporate strength training exercises at least twice a week to help maintain muscle mass and improve insulin sensitivity.

**Monitoring and Medication**

- 11. Blood Sugar Monitoring: Regularly monitor your blood sugar levels to understand how different foods and activities affect them

- 12. Medication Adherence: Take your diabetes medications or insulin as prescribed by your healthcare provider.

**Lifestyle Changes**

- 13. Weight Management: Maintain a healthy weight to improve blood sugar control and reduce the risk of complications.

- 14. **Stress Management:** Practice stress-reducing activities such as meditation, yoga, or deep-breathing exercises.

- 15. **Quit Smoking:** If you smoke, seek help to quit as smoking can increase the risk of diabetes complications.

- 16. **Limit Alcohol:** Drink alcohol in moderation, if at all, and always with food.

**Sleep and Routine**

- 17. **Adequate Sleep:** Ensure you get 7-8 hours of quality sleep each night to help regulate blood sugar levels.

- 18. **Consistent Routine:** Maintain a consistent daily routine for meals, exercise, and medication.

**Education and Support**

- 19. **Education:** Stay informed about diabetes management through reliable sources and educational programs.

- 20. **Support System:** Build a support system of family, friends, and healthcare professionals to help manage diabetes effectively.

These tips can help manage diabetes and improve overall health and well-being.

*Dear Readers,*

*I want to extend my heartfelt gratitude to each one of you for taking the time to read my book. Your support and interest mean the world to me. Whether you are new to the world of managing diabetes or have been on this journey for a while, I hope you found the tips and advice helpful and empowering.*

*Your health and well-being are incredibly important, and it is my sincere hope that this book has provided you with valuable insights and practical strategies to manage diabetes effectively. Remember, every small step you take towards a healthier lifestyle is a significant achievement.*

*Thank you for being a part of this journey with me. Your feedback and support are greatly appreciated and inspire me to continue creating content that can make a positive impact.*

*Wishing you all the best on your path to health and happiness.*

*Warm regards,*

## Author's

Growing up in the heart of the South, I was surrounded by the rich, comforting flavors of soul food. From family gatherings to Sunday dinners, soul food was more than just a meal; it was a way to bring people together, to celebrate life, and to create lasting memories. However, my journey took an unexpected turn when I was diagnosed with type 2 diabetes. Suddenly, the foods I had always cherished became a source of concern.

Determined not to let diabetes define me or take away the joy of eating, I embarked on a mission to reinvent soul food in a way that was both delicious and diabetes-friendly. This cookbook is the culmination of years of research, experimentation, and personal experience. It's my hope that these recipes will help others enjoy the flavors they love while maintaining a healthy lifestyle.

## Dedication

This book is dedicated to my family, who have been my biggest supporters and taste-testers throughout this journey. To my mother, who taught me the basics of soul food cooking, and to my children, who inspire me to create healthier versions of our favorite dishes.

## Acknowledgements

*I would like to express my deepest gratitude to the following individuals and organizations:*

- My Family and Friends: Thank you for your unwavering support and encouragement. Your love and patience have been invaluable.

- Recipe Testers: Thank you to the friends and volunteers who tested countless recipes, providing feedback and suggestions to perfect each dish.

- Publishers and Editors: I am immensely grateful for your expertise and dedication in bringing this cookbook to life. Your hard work has made this project possible.

- Photographers and Designers: Your talent and creativity have captured the essence of these dishes, making this cookbook visually appealing and inviting.

- Readers and Supporters: To everyone who has supported this journey, thank you. Your encouragement and shared stories have been a source of motivation and inspiration.

***This cookbook is a labor of love, created with the hope of making a positive impact on the lives of those managing diabetes. It is a testament to the idea that with determination and creativity, we can transform challenges into opportunities for growth and enjoyment. Enjoy these recipes, savor the flavors, and remember that a diabetes diagnosis is not the end, but a new beginning to a healthier, more flavorful life.***